DYSLEXIA

How do we learn?

DYSLEXIA

How do we learn?

John O'Shea & Jenny Dalton
with Doris Zagdanski

Hill of Content

First published in Australia 1994
by Hill of Content Publishing Company Pty Ltd
86 Bourke Street, Melbourne, Australia 3000

© Copyright John O'Shea 1994

Typeset by Midland Typesetters, Maryborough, Victoria.
Design: Guy Mirabella
Printed in Australia by Australian Print Group, Maryborough, Victoria.

National Library of Australia
Cataloguing-in-Publication data

O'Shea, John 1966–
 Dyslexia: how do we learn?

 ISBN 0 85572 236 3

 1. Dyslexia. 2. Learning Disabilities. 3. Dyslexics—education.
 I. Dalton, Jenny, 1950– . II. Zagdanski, Doris, 1954– .
 III. Title.

371.9144

Audio tape available from The Royal Institute for the Blind Talking Book Library, 85 High Street, Prahran 3181.
Tel. (03) 521 3400, (008) 33 5588.

Contents

Introduction vi

Part 1
John's Story 1

Part 2
A Case Study 41

Part 3
How to Help 67

References 105

Additional reading 107

Index 109

Introduction

Have you ever felt like you would rather go fishing than go to school? I have. There were many times when I would replace my books with fishing tackle and a change of clothes, knowing full well what the consequences would be, but chose to do it anyway. The fun outweighed the risk of punishment and the risk of punishment was nothing in comparison with my fear of the classroom.

This is one side of my story—a bit of adventure, wagging, playing hookey, outwitting parents and teachers. The other side is about walking into an English lesson knowing I would have to read aloud and feel sick in my stomach, having butterflies and sweaty palms, and ending up in the toilet crying. All because I couldn't read.

I don't have a disease or a physical deformity but what I do have is a very real and common problem that I share with many other individuals. From the time I started school I lived with the thought of being useless and dumb when it came to writing, spelling and communication. No one seemed to understand the problem and no one really wanted anything to do with it.

The only time there was any relief for me was when I was doing sport or any other activity which took me out of the classroom. I was good at sport—not because I was gifted or had private lessons but because I never had to use my brain, or at least it didn't feel like a great effort, when I was doing sport. Sometimes I felt like my head didn't belong to my body and often I thought that it had been sewn on to the wrong person!

So why would a dyslexic person like me want to write a book? After all, I have spent the greater part of my life trying to avoid reading. I even think it's ironic that here I am writing an introduction when I've never even read one!

I want to begin by telling you where the idea of this book came from. It all started in 1990 when I confronted my literacy problem and decided to do something about it. I was dissatisfied with the way my reading and writing skills had not developed even after spending most of my life at school. The thought of writing a letter was a nightmare, a thank you note was an impossibility and leaving a message on the door for a friend was embarrassing.

It was suggested that I contact Jenny Dalton, a teacher who worked in the Learning Skills Unit at the Gordon Technical College, Geelong. One of the first questions Jenny asked me was how did I learn. Straight away I knew this was my chance to learn my way. I had already explained that I wanted to improve my reading and writing but I didn't want to go back to all the useless exercises I'd done at school for so many years.

Over time, we developed my personal dictionary, using words from my own writing as I wrote about subjects which were of interest to me. Eventually we even spent time on the unforgiving rules of English which, for the first time, seemed to make sense and stick in my head.

Slowly I was beginning to feel confident to tackle tasks which before I thought were impossible. I was no longer alone and fighting a battle that I could not win. The desire to write about my school experiences started as a good way for me to be motivated to write for the sake of writing. It developed into a passion that I could not stop. Jenny continually encouraged, corrected and encouraged more.

The thought of confronting my biggest social and personal problem became more exciting than powder skiing in France. The challenge ran deep and my fear was great, but the desire to succeed was even greater. There was so much I wanted to write about. It was as if I had not been able to talk and all of a sudden someone granted me the use of words.

John O'Shea

Part 1

John's Story

Background
When he first approached me to inquire about help with his reading and writing, John was adamant that he wanted none of the strategies to which he had been subjected as a child. He had failed them all. And they had failed him.

I didn't want to read their stupid books to start with ... I was into sport and all these things. For me, the process of learning to read wasn't about Pat and Ben—so why couldn't I read something I enjoyed reading? I never read any books through the whole of school.

Being labelled as a dyslexic at a young age is no easy thing to fight off in the playground. 'Here comes Brains', the kids used to say.

I began with the suggestion that John should try writing about himself and his childhood experiences. This had a somewhat cathartic effect as he recalled and explored the events that had brought him as a confident, articulate 25 year old, with a tertiary level education qualification, to seek help with his reading and writing.

As John's stories developed, I became increasingly intrigued by the patterns that were emerging: the early signs of school problems, the increasingly futile and even counter-productive attempts to 'help' him with his school work, the frustration, bad behaviour and distress that evolved and overriding all of this, his strong belief in his own knowledge of himself.

The extent of the writing and the quality of the information it contained, suggested a value that went beyond the immediate function of encouraging him to write. The search for an understanding of Dyslexia through the lived experience of someone like John has brought a depth of reality to the subject which is not evident through the more theoretical, scientific studies of the subject that are available. John's recollections have illuminated the *moments of crisis* that have occurred in his life and through this means it is possible for us to view his experience from within.

John refers to himself as 'dyslexic' and uses the term 'dyslexia' to refer to the difficulties he has experienced in learning how to read and write. Used in this way, 'dyslexia' is a useful term because it literally means:

dys—*having difficulty with*
lexia—*the language*

However, we need to be wary of using it to mean

anything more than that. Here in Australia, there has been a reluctance to even use the term, because of the dangers that are perceived in so labelling people. It is a very controversial subject and there are many theories which attempt to explain why some, otherwise capable, intelligent people, seem to experience such difficulties with written language. Unfortunately there are no clearcut answers or explanations.

So the terms 'dyslexia' and 'dyslexic' in these pages are used simply as a shorthand way of saying 'having difficulty with learning certain skills of language'. Use of the term does not mean an endorsement of any particular theory associated with the causes of such difficulties.

John identified the goals associated with this writing project as follows:

- To give people with literacy difficulties encouragement to have faith in themselves; especially young people and to stress the importance of working at the things they are good at.
- To encourage teachers to treat the class as individuals and to look for strategies that will work for individuals.
- To enable people to know what it is like to be 'on the other side', in other words to be unable to read and write.
- To give families encouragement.

Having embarked upon this project, he generated a large amount of written anecdotal material related to his learning history. Some of the stories are humorous in the case of pranks he got up to in his never-ending struggle to assert his power over those who seemed intent on bringing him down; others were sad or poignant as he described the battles he waged in order to maintain his sense of himself.

The effect of this writing was to prompt him early in the process to note:

I have confidence in an area that I always looked upon as a handicap. People often say they have one great handicap. This to me was a life long sentence into a world that I would never know the other side of English. Now some of the complex English there seems so basic ... my desire is so strong like a dog on the scent of a fox chase. I have the taste of success in my mouth. A true need to improve on my weakness. The self pride and satisfaction of being able to express myself with the pen.

Clearly with this project John was able to enter a new dimension in his attitude to writing. On his first attempt he wrote:

The galaciy of Dislecsia

I really feel good about the throught of wrtting a book or some nots on a problem which I have. Maybe I can help some easle, mabe I can help myself. Comint to turms with personal problems is never easy, but coming toraillty about this problon I have is almost impossible.

Im the normal kid in class, I have nothing extrat to offer and No really speacial skills in the envronment they call learning. Infact I hate learning and the class room so much ... Fustraction would be on of the biggest effect I have, the understand even the knowlage, but not the ability to exspress it or read it.

I have only written two very small pages in this old diary I have and allready I feel this great sence of achivement. I now don't care if I never see my words on a book shelf or in the best sellars list. I just feel fantastic about the challange and the feelong that I really want to do this.

My mind know thinks that if I'm going to do this I must do it well. Show myself can do it and if some day you end up reading it you will see Hay that block could really do something if he putts his mind to it.

A deeply held desire to succeed and enormous excitement were generated at the prospect of beginning to write freely. This was particularly so in relation to his fantasy about becoming a writer. It was from this acknowledgement of his dream of being a writer (and not only a writer but obviously one who could thumb his nose at those who would interpret dyslexia as a sign of ineptitude) that the idea emerged in his mind to collect the pieces he had written together into a book.

Jenny Dalton

1

What's wrong with me? I have two arms, two legs, all the parts of my body are in the right place and I can see with perfect vision. So, from the outside, I look okay. But I'm dyslexic. This means I have problems with the normal process of learning. On the inside, in my head, something I don't fully understand happens when I try to read or write.

If you ask someone what they think dyslexia is, I'm sure you would get replies which sound something like this:

Dyslexia is a reading and writing problem.

You get things back to front.

The page moves when you read.

You have learning difficulties.

Your brain malfunctions.

Of course all of these things could be true and there are often associated problems as well. For me, dyslexia is both simpler and yet more complicated. The simple part is that the words do appear back to front when I read and they never stand still on a page. But the awful part about dyslexia is what it does to your self esteem. At school I was made to feel useless and stupid. I found school hard from Day One and the feeling of having to go back, day after day, was very hard. I felt that I was guilty of some great crime and to be sent to school was my punishment.

But my only crime was that I had problems with reading and writing. Often I would leave words out of a sentence but when I read the work back to myself I would not notice anything missing. This made my stories disjointed.

When I'd sit down to read only one word stood still on the page and the others decided to have a party. Within a matter of minutes I would become nauseous. Not sick or feeling like I was going to throw up my lunch, but more like being car sick. It's hard to explain, but it is not easy to read or concentrate when this happens. Have you ever tried to read in the car, and you start to feel a little sick, well that is almost the feeling.

The reason I say almost is because not only is there the feeling of being sick, the words are all going in different directions. Try to imagine only seeing one word at a time and all the words around it are going in a circular motion. It's damn hard to get any rhythm or fluency with your reading when it's like this. So it's almost as if I know the words that are in front of me but, because I'm so slow in working them out and concentrating extra hard, after reading two or three pages I cannot remember a word I've read.

It's a bit like when you've been driving a car for a long time and you're tired and the road starts to blend into a continuous blur. Well this is what it's like when I read but it starts from the minute I get behind the wheel of a book.

When I write, I'd put my letters back to front or I'd read them backwards. Most of the time I had no idea I was even doing it. Another trick my eyes would play was that I would see only half a word—but it didn't matter. I would guess the word that I thought should go there; often I'd be right but sometimes I would come up with some doozies!

We can sometimes see something in front of us, but not understand what it is or recognise its purpose. Often I felt like this at school. School work was like a huge mirage, vivid and clear, yet as soon as I got closer to it, it would vanish in front of me.

I really enjoy skiing in a whiteout; it's better if it's a clear day and the snow is fresh. Skiing in a whiteout is great for your skiing because you are unable to see and must rely on feeling through your feet and body. It's as if you have your eyes open, yet can't see, but you are still able to do the task required.

School work paints the same vivid picture of getting to the end of a problem and not being able to understand how or why you got the result you did—but you got there. When I could not understand what I had done yesterday it was damned hard to repeat it the next day. I would often spell the same word three or four different ways on the one page. I recently heard that Benjamin Franklin once said that an educated man should be able to spell any word at least six ways! But teachers could never understand why I could do it yesterday, and today I had to start all over again. Skiing blind in a blizzard and going to school often feel the same to me, but skiing is a lot easier than school work ever was.

I hated English most of all. That's when my fears and failures were put on display for the whole class to see. What I dreaded most was being asked to read aloud in front of everyone.

And it wasn't only the reading. The lead up was just as bad. When I knew it was getting closer to my turn the sweaty palms would start. I'd get nervous, agitated. Often I'd watch the clock to see how many minutes were left in the lesson, hoping the bell would ring before my turn. Or else I'd insist I had to go to the toilet—any excuse to escape the humiliation.

2

School to me was like a train track and planned to the last full stop. By Grade X you were meant to have learnt so much and so on. Well I'm an individual and I felt as though the whole class was rushing past me. I felt like taking a detour and stopping for a while to see if the traffic would slow down. But before I knew it I was in 6th grade, being told I have the skills of 3rd grade and the train was still moving along those tracks and it never slowed down or stopped so I could get back on board. The other kids all seemed like they were progressing but not me, I was on a train ride to hell.

It was like a group of bush walkers going up a hill. Those in front stop to wait for the others who aren't as fast. The ones who wait have an opportunity to rest, drink some water and get their breath back. But as soon as the others arrive they're off again. So the back people never really get a rest at all and become slower and slower. And those in front become faster.

Being a rebel or a disturbance in class became a necessity for me. In junior school my nickname was 'Trouble' and later it changed to 'Brains'. At times I felt so inadequate that if I didn't do something, I thought I might explode. I can always remember feeling so useless and stupid, because deep down I knew all the answers but I just couldn't work them out or write them down. I had built up such a negative feeling about myself that before long the most basic things became impossible.

I was catching a disease more dangerous than dyslexia; I was becoming scared to learn. I had very low self esteem and a mental picture that I was useless. I felt a huge amount of anger and I think this anger has been the reason for my survival. Many teachers said I was lazy and others would say I could do the work if I only tried harder. But in both cases it didn't seem to work and the more I tried, the blanker my brain went.

In the endeavour of trying to do everything right, my parents had me tested, analysed and categorised for the benefit of themselves and the school. Looking back I often question the intentions of making me look at ink blots and stupid puzzles. I am not saying that they do not help parents and teachers to have a greater understanding of where your limitations are, but you must realise that the student feels like he or she has a disease. In my case, all the tests and all the prodding and even the coloured glasses from America did not improve my reading or writing.

From Grade 3 I would continually have extra

English or tutors to assist with my problem. This could have been of great advantage as far as my learning was concerned but it had disastrous effects on me personally and socially. At times I would grasp the meanings in the extra English classes and feel that I was going forward, but the damage that was caused by my friends or the others in the playground meant that the benefits were soon lost.

Because the school had its boundaries and limitations in regard to flexibility, the majority of my extra English or remedial classes, as they were called, were done at times to suit the school or the family unit. These times were either prior to my first class early in the morning or immediately after school. Both times never really suited me, and I would have much preferred to have been playing with my friends after or before school instead of having to regurgitate the same English, the same difficulties and the same lack of understanding during this time.

I remember especially one night sitting in bed trying to read some English text out loud to my mother, continually struggling with every word and not grasping the meanings or themes the book was trying to convey. In frustration and anger I began to cry. For the next hour my mother held me and she too was crying. Throughout my senior years I found that I was lost in a world that made no sense to me. I had been tested, re-tested and analysed yet there was no clear answer or visual picture that explained why the words had a 'party' on the page while I was trying to read.

So I decided to excel at being a class disturbance. I had more detentions than cut lunches! As I grew older and my reading and writing stagnated, my devious exploits grew and expanded into areas that even surprised me. While the other students worked I would often spend the day testing the limitations of my teachers!

What I did learn was that ultimately I would never win in these encounters so that's when I became serious. Again I see (and saw) this as a survival mechanism. So instead of confronting a situation and knowing I was going to lose, regardless of whether it was my fault or a misunderstanding, I would creatively look for ways around the situation.

One of my devious techniques was confusion. Or playing dumb. I loved to deliver psychological blows to my opponents; I could point out where their weaknesses lay and my strength lay in being able to withstand the pressure to confess. There is no doubt that I broke the rules but rarely could they pin it on me.

Once there was the 'blue-tack on the bell' incident. At the end of each meal, one of the masters on duty would pick up the hand bell and ring it loudly to signal quiet for general announcements. As the master rose from his high position at the top table most of the diners would be aware that it was time for announcements and they would turn towards him. So, on this occasion, with at least 180 pairs of eyes on him (including mine), he proceeded to 'ring' the bell, but of course nothing happened and the laughter started and rapidly filled the hall. If you have all those kids laughing at you—it's not all that funny, so of course the issue then became finding the culprit and that's when the real fun began for me.

I was the only one who knew who had put the bluetack in the bell. It was not important to me to impress the other students so I had no need to prewarn my mates. I enjoyed immensely watching the frustration of the teacher as he attempted to find the culprit. His aggression in this situation was no different to mine. The frustration was the same—now he knew what it felt like. This would also extend to the rest of the school because once he had exhausted all his strategies he would threaten the whole school with punishment unless the culprit owned up. Then the students would start looking around, myself included, to see who had done it. As there was no pressure from my table because no one knew it was me, I could enjoy it even more.

I should add in defence of my honour that if it ever got to the point of everyone being punished I would own up because by then I'd had my fun.

And what could they do anyway? The usual punishment was to have to run!! I loved it. But there is no doubt that if the cane had still been in use I would have thought twice about my crimes—at my primary school I had had experience of six layers of leather doused in vinegar and the memory of the pain remains with me.

Here's another incident of a similar nature. One master owned a dog which would often come into class. One day I used my left hand (which wasn't all that much different to my right hand actually) to write an abusive letter attacking this particular teacher and signed it from his dog and then attached it to the dog. When the dog arrived at class, as he always did, I remember the teacher saying, 'And what have they stuck on you?' and he removed it and read it.

My pleasure in this incident came from his total lack of response. He showed absolutely no emotion and to my mind this would have been very difficult for him. He was a very inquisitive sort of person and had to know everything. I'm sure he knew that it was me, and he knew that I knew that he knew and that there was absolutely nothing he could do. He was an ex policeman and fully aware of the need for proof—and he had none. Once again I identify this with my own feelings at report time—that struggle to appear calm, composed and unaffected by what was written—I enjoyed watching him go through that struggle.

If I felt that if people respected me I would do anything for them. I would crawl over an acre of broken glass for them. But if they treated me like a stupid moron I would lose respect for them. I was always taught to have enormous respect for my elders—and at times I still feel that this is important, but now this must be accompanied by them giving me respect. This did not happen at school so in my mind I was not being rude or disrespectful.

When I felt I was losing control of my situation, the only way I knew how to survive was to become aggressive. I don't really like that word—I prefer to think I was angry and stubborn with frustration. But my teachers called it aggression. I'll admit I could use cutting remarks that were always very direct. My language could be colourful too and I had no hesitation in swearing at a teacher. I did it because I felt provoked. The frustration I had been feeling throughout most of my schooling would just spill over and my remarks or reactions often carried with them years of accumulated hurt, confusion, tension and embarrassment.

To them 'mobile disaster' would be an understatement. But I was more than just a disturbance. I baffled them with my learning problems as well. So they put me in the too-hard basket and I always ended up at the bottom of the pile. Like when they graded us according to our ability and I was put in 'G' set. The best students were in 'A' set, 'B' set was for the next best and so on. Even I knew that G came after A, B, C, D, E, and F. When you spend your life in 'G' set, you start to believe all the negative things about yourself and by the time your maturity catches up with you you've been left behind.

The only time I got a B grading for a subject was for Physical Education. All my other results were always D or E. But what got to me the most was that even when I did try my hardest they still failed me. All they would look at was my spelling and writing—they never gave me any credit for the effort.

I couldn't believe it when my final P.E. report said,

He put in the effort but was not up to the general standard in his written work.
Spelling really held him back.

Imagine putting a whole year's work into something you loved, only to be told that you had failed! It was an area of school that I totally enjoyed, yet failed. The thing I most wanted to be was a Physical Education teacher and I had just failed Fifth Form in that subject as well as the others.

Over the years my school reports reinforced the entire situation:

John does not appear to have much confidence in his own ability and his extrovert manner in class does not disguise this.

He has been impetuous, restless and disoriented.

Crashed abysmally in the examination paper

Something of a hazard in the laboratory.

Concentration span is very limited.

You may find these reports gloomy.

Huge fluctuations in mood and behaviour.

I know he is capable of better attainment.

Both distracts and is distracted.

Then after all the hassles of the past years, there came the grand finale—my Form 5 (Year 11) report. This was the final cruncher.

Every year, report time was the same at our house. I would sit in the loungeroom waiting for my father to get home with my report sitting in front of me. Mum would have already opened it and had a look. I'd often ask was it good or how did I go and invariably she would say something like, 'Not that crash hot but you can wait till your father comes home to discuss it.'

For me it was like a Tattslotto ticket that you presume is going to be a loser but you always hope that maybe this one will be a winner. In my mind there'd be pictures of scholarships, streamers, balloons, chocolate cake and all the things that mark a reward for effort.

This was an annual ritual—mum would confirm that the report was bad so I would reluctantly retire to the loungeroom to read the reports from the battlefield and see how many casualties there were. This was not easy because of the handwriting styles of the enemy—they might as well have been writing in Morse code. But I always understood what the bottom line was.

In our house you can hear the car drive into the drive way and I was never sure just how long I would have to wait for the 'discussion'. There was usually a feeling of wanting to get out of there because it seemed that I had no avenues of escape from the teachers' reports—they were never wrong and this was especially the case when they were all clearly in conspiracy with each other. I knew I would have to draw on all my skills of creativity and imagination in order to explain what I saw as their lack of understanding of my problem.

As I sat waiting I could feel the anxiety building up; it wasn't that I was afraid of punishment, it was more related to the disappointment that I would be causing. I felt that I was letting down everyone in the family because my sister and brother never had reports like mine. There was no sense of satisfaction for me in this, no pleasure to be found in being different.

I should point out that my dad and I are very similar except that now I'm taller—we have similar mannerisms, language, voice tone, colouring and these days my mother often can't tell us apart on the phone. Our communication normally is very friendly and we have a great rapport. But this was one of the times when things were different. I knew that when he came in, he would look stern and sound strong and confident. If I was sitting in his chair, instead of greeting me with the usual sarcastic, 'Are you comfortable there?' it would be, 'Get out of my chair—this is not going to be pretty'. He would sometimes remind us that we had opportunities that he'd never had and that we seemed to take for granted the effort he put in at work in order to supply us with our education and family needs.

As I sat there, I would hear the familiar sound of him arriving home—and at that point my heart would start to race, my palms would instantly become sweaty and enormous effort would go into appearing calm. I would know the action was about to start so I would adopt a very poker faced look—not sad, not scared, not sorry.

From the Housemaster
December 15th 1982

Dear Brian and Naomi,

John's academic results will be a disappointment to him. He has worked hard this term and there has been a considerable improvement in most subject areas. The unpalatable fact has to be faced, namely that John does not have the ability to reach the standard that this school requires for a Form Five (Year 11) pass in most subjects. In your letter to his teachers you asked that he be given 'a fair go in regard to his ability and given as much encouragement as possible'. I am pleased to say that this has been done and he has at last realised that being a nuisance in class is totally unproductive.

Professor C. in his two reports that you have kindly sent me states that John should be able to make progress at a secondary school until Form Five level and that he should then make an occupational choice which is appropriate for his interests and abilities. He also states that he ought to attempt year 12 at a school that has an alternative Year 12 Programme.

There would seem to be three options open. First, he should come back to repeat his Form Five year in totality. I doubt very much that the results at the end of 1983 would be vastly different from those of 1982. He would also find it difficult to select seven subjects that would hold his interest. Secondly, he could attempt the new mixed course that I have spoken about. Here he would only have to do three Form Five subjects and there would be scope for general education. By this means he might manage to secure a so-called pass at Leaving, but we must ask ourselves to what end this pass is aimed. He is not going to be able to cope with tertiary education on any scale at all. Unfortunately his grades would seem to preclude this option.

The third alternative is probably the most sensible from an academic point of view. He should leave school and continue his studies part time whilst undertaking some course or training as suggested by Professor C. I fully realise that he is young to leave school and we must face the facts of his ability and his potential. He is not likely to make much academic progress here but he might, hopefully, make some progress in other areas.

As you know he has caused a great deal of trouble in the past few weeks. As I mentioned earlier in the letter he has now stopped being a nuisance in class but his behaviour to some masters had been most objectionable. At his best, he is keen, helpful and *well mannered. At his worst he is aggressive, rude and devious.*

When we have spoken recently about the various occurrences involving John, you have asked me to give him the benefit of the doubt in certain cases. It must be realised quite clearly that in some cases there is no doubt at all. He cut Chapel knowing that he had to attend. He was rude to the House Captain who was only doing his duty by telling him to wear a tie. His study was dirty despite several warnings from me. He did receive remarkable, in my view, consideration in the incident involving a Middle School boy and he did not initially tell the whole truth about the incident. I have given him the benefit of the doubt over the repeated use of his study by boarders at the weekend, but I must admit that I now doubt the wisdom of my judgement as I have been told, perhaps wrongly and maliciously, that John and / or Matthew left their key with some boarders from time to time.

Anyhow all the above is past history. I am more than willing to forget the past and welcome him back here next year but I must make myself absolutely clear on one vital point. He returns to my House on the School's terms. I shall not allow him or anyone else to cause such disruptions as John and others have caused this year. He has told me that he does not like my choice of prefects for 1983 and that he does not like the way that I run the House. He is naturally perfectly entitled to those opinions.

If he is to have a successful year he has got to learn to live with authority. If he is willing to do that then

I shall be only too happy to have him back again. He has a lot to offer in many fields.

Happy Christmas.

The opening line said my reports will be a 'disappointment'. What an understatement! I had failed every subject in my final year. In addition there were graphic examples of my 'aggressive', 'rude', and 'devious' exploits during the year. I was doomed. Happy Christmas—what a joke!

3

The headmaster wrote that the 'unpalatable fact' had to be faced that I did not have the ability to reach the standard that this school requires 'for a Form Five (Year 11) pass in most subjects'.

The key word here is *ability*. I maintain that he didn't know what my ability was because he had never tapped into it. To me it was a reminder of the round pegs and square holes that I had been given to play around with when I was much younger. What he said was probably right in terms of that school—no doubt I would not meet their requirements but the implication was, both here and through the rest of the report, that the fault lay very much with me rather than with the school. I believe that we both contributed to the problem.

This report quotes Professor C. who concludes that basically I was a dyslexic retard. Now let me fill you in a little on the Professor. This guy was the leading professor in this field and he was going to 'shine the light on all my problems'. My parents had been referred to this expert by a number of people such as the careers teacher and others at the school. His establishment was old and unimpressive and he was very much of the old school. He seemed old to me and looked down over his glasses at me.

His advice was of great reassurance to my parents but as usual I felt completely out of the picture. To my mind the consultation did nothing for me. For a start I didn't know what he was doing. What seemed like an endless parade of ink blots that looked like butterflies left me cold. What the hell was I meant to do?

Mum and Dad would be waiting out in the waiting room—this was meant to be my big chance. This was where we would all find out where the fault lay—what was causing the rattle—a bit like getting your car serviced really, when you find out what is causing the problem you don't tell the car you tell the owner and that's what it felt like. While I performed the various tests he would sit writing down things that I couldn't see.

The tests seemed endless—I remember things like a picture of someone cutting a hedge and there was a car sitting on top of the hedge instead of being in the car park.

When he asked me to explain what was happening in the picture I would deliberately ignore the fact that the house had no roof or the car was parked on the hedge and say something like: 'the guy is cutting the hedge from left to right and he should be going right to left', or something to that effect.

I remember that he would flash a card with a picture quite quickly and then I'd have to remember what I had seen in order to explain it. But this was easy for me—it was no different to when mum used to put things out in the kitchen and then take some away and I would have to say what had been removed. I've got a good visual memory.

When I had finished performing I was sent out to wait while my parents were called back in. It makes me think now of people at an audition. They have the spotlight focused on them and everyone else is in the darkness beyond the stage—the only feedback they get when they finish is—'we'll call you'. So they're left wondering whether they had been any good or not.

At the time I had a strong feeling that I should have been included in those discussions. I am sure that my parents would have filled me in on some of the things that were said but it is not the same as being there as a participant in the room. After all, it was me that had the problem and not them.

While I feel that the professor's processes were impersonal his analysis was quite correct. He said that I should be able to make it to Form 5 (Year 11) at a secondary school but then I would need to make an 'occupational choice' based on my interests and abilities and that an alternative Year 12 would need to be found. He was almost right except that in actual fact I didn't even pass at Form 5!

The Professor had helped my parents by reassuring them that the problem could be labelled, boxed and categorised, and he had helped the teachers come to the conclusion that I had no potential and there was no place for me in this school.

So I changed schools. This time it was a government state school which was trialling a new Year 12 course called Tertiary Orientation Program (T.O.P.) This course was different because students undertook goal based assessment projects rather than the usual 3 hour final exam.

In a paper published by the Victorian Association for the Teaching of English, my new English teacher wrote:

There is one way in which assessment can be used to benefit students through its actual process. I discovered it through teaching English B, where assessment is 'continuous, diagnostic and participatory', and I wish that every English teacher could have the opportunity to experience, just once, what this means in practice and feel the intrinsic joy and satisfaction that it brings for teacher and students alike.

The most immediately noticeable difference in the assessment process of English B is the absence of an external examination. This departure is greeted by students with a deep sense of liberation, but there is a profound fear in the minds of most teachers that once the barrier of the external examination is removed laziness and mediocrity will sprawl unchecked, standards will drop, individual excellence will wither away and the subject English itself will be utterly and irretrievably demeaned. I would like to try to allay some of these fears by describing what actually happens to a group of Year 12 students from whom the threat—or spur—of an external examination has been removed.

The first thing I noticed amongst them as I said, was a buoyant feeling of relief, expressed in terms of such intensity that I was forced to realise fully, for the first time, how crippling the prospect of an external examination is for many students. One student wrote,

'As the crowd gathered around the door and all the year's work was riding on my shoulders, I felt the enormous pressure of the examination. Everyone was chattering when the huge doors opened and then a nervous hush came over the room and over me. The rules were read out to us and then the race was on. It was like the start to a marathon and I was stuck to my seat. I felt the whole room rush past me and I was dumbfounded.'[1.]

That student was me.
This is what else my English teacher had to say:

Every student in the group was new to me. Each one had been unsatisfied by their previous achievements in English classes. This subject offered a new freedom—as long as clearly stated writing goals were met, and specific tasks completed, we could choose our topics from a rich array of interests and ideas. I had a feeling that in this group, ideas would pop into focus like light bulbs at the flick of a switch.

The group was small enough to squash round a large table in one of the conference rooms in the school library. Just working in a circle, instead of the gritty, uncompromising rows of classroom desks made a difference. There was something special, too, about the newness of the subject—we all felt that the spotlight was on us—it was our responsibility to show how well it could work. And my personal goal was to show every member of the group that they could be, not just efficient writers, but good writers.

At the end of the first session, John stayed behind to tell me that he had a great deal of difficulty with reading. He asked me not to call on him to read aloud. He described his difficulties in such a straightforward way that I was inclined to disregard what he told me as an exaggeration, or perhaps a lack of confidence. How could such an articulate student be unable to read? John appeared to be such a competent student that I was unable to take in the clear message that he was giving me. It was only later that I realised how much effort it must have cost him to make that statement to me.

I also realised later how privileged I was to receive the information. John found himself unable to make the same statement to his drama teacher, and resorted instead to slipping out of sight when drama classes were on. This strategy soon resulted in what was for me a very puzzling parent teacher meeting. I sat there listening to the drama teacher (usually a very gentle man) as he angrily complained about John's uncooperative behaviour. Could this be my best student? I defended him as well as I could, astonished by the drama teacher's uncharacteristic behaviour.

My belief in John's capability was so strong that it could easily have become counter productive, even damaging. Because I was so convinced that John was exaggerating his inability to read, I blithely forgot about his request after the first few weeks and routinely included him in oral reading activities. Nothing about John's performance reminded me of our conversation. He seemed to manage extremely well. He might have stumbled occasionally, but so did everyone else. How did he do it?

One of the texts which we worked with that year was Tom Stoppard's play. In my diary for that year I found this entry: 'we started Inspector Hound today. All we could do was laugh.' I think perhaps that the enjoyment we all shared must have provided some sort of psychological uplift which buffered the students against failure. Maybe it was a bit like tightrope walking—the readers just kept on showing their skills, held upright by a thin thread of exuberance.

John explains it now simply by saying that when he was asked to read, he made up his own words. And yet, at the time, I was following the text carefully, and didn't pick up any inconsistencies.

Another experience which boosted the confidence of the group was cross age tutoring. My Year 7 English class was about to start on a story writing activity, and I suggested that the English B students might like to teach them how. After an initial attack of misgivings, they agreed. From the start of the first 'getting to know you' session, they established excellent working relationships with their Year 7 partners. It was delightful to see the caring teaching which took place. As the English B students struggled to clarify the goals and explain the processes of short story writing to their Year 7 students, their own understanding and confidence blossomed. The comments of the Year 7 students at the end of the programme reflected their enthusiasm and appreciation. One student wrote, 'it was good fun working with John. He had more time to spend with us.'

Amongst all the happy memories of that year, however, the one that sparkles most for me is the memory of the Sportsmen's Dinner.

One of the most exciting parts of the English B course was the Production Unit, which allowed each student to complete a project of their own choice. This unit of work was a challenging one; it demanded careful forward planning, organisation, and a certain amount of vision and enthusiasm. John and three other boys decided to do something to help unemployed young people. Their discussions focused on a fundraising activity, and they finally decided to hold a Sportsmens' Dinner at the Geelong Football Club.

As I watched them designing tickets, making phone calls, organising publicity, arranging for catering, managing interviews, writing letters to sponsors and attending to hundreds of other necessary tasks, they seemed to grow before my eyes into confident young men.

The night was a magical success. I doubt if John will ever forget it. When John led the speakers in the door I knew that all those months of hard work had been worthwhile. One of the boys wrote later in his evaluation report, 'It is still difficult to understand how a group of students could organise such an evening'. But they did.

At last someone had recognised it. I wasn't dumb. I could learn but not by reading books or writing things down. Instead I learn by doing. I am a do-er.

No doubt about it, I was different; I didn't understand the writing on the blackboard, and I couldn't do dictation. But I'm not stupid and schools shouldn't have boxed me into the slow learning group. I should have been put into an area which allowed me to learn with great speed and understanding,—the DO-ERS' CLASS.

4

I learn by doing. I learn by feeling what is happening to me. I don't remember things by writing them down—I remember by visualizing what is going on around me and then recalling the places, people, stories and experiences along the way.

I've travelled overseas but I can't read the names of the places I have visited. However, I can give you a blow by blow description of what they look like, how the people act and what they do, because I have seen them and felt what it was like to live there. I remember having no trouble learning how to drive but I failed the written test. At school I was disadvantaged whenever I was in the classroom but not when I was outside doing sport. I can ski, rock climb, paddle grade five rapids and pick up almost any sport on sight. It was this ability to *do*, not read or write, which eventually helped me to pass my final year at school.

Trish, a friend of my brother's, and a Phys. Ed.

major at university, volunteered to help me study for my exams. While I just sat staring at my books knowing that all this stuff wouldn't sink in, she noticed my frustration. She then asked me how did I learn.

At first I was not sure what she meant. No one had ever asked me this before, but my reply was the reason I passed the exams at the end of the year ... *I learn by doing.* So she suggested we go down to the beach and by the time we got there I had explained my answer in detail, and the learning was about to start, my way.

The rest of the weekend I didn't have to open a book or write one word. We played tennis, went swimming, ran along the beach and studied. While we played tennis we would talk non stop about all aspects of P.E. Every time I made a move or did something I had to describe the action, or explain the muscle used. Trish was teaching me all the things I had tried to read but found so hard to understand. It was fantastic, not only was I understanding, I could remember it. For the very first time in my life something so difficult was becoming second nature.

Then in the exam room I went through all the same procedures to recall the information I'd learned at the beach. I'd stand up and swing my arm to remember the names of the muscles—I know it gave everyone else the willies but what the heck, I passed!

Although my dreams were to be a P.E. teacher, I ended up gaining a place at Bendigo College to study Outdoor Education. My final exam results, with special consideration in the marking and a successful interview helped to get me there.

Since then I have been a ski instructor, mountain guide in the high country, lived with the Aboriginals in Northern Territory, worked as a private nurse in England, and I have renovated the house I live in. Although my love and passion is the great outdoors, I now find myself a manager and salesperson in my family's business.

Have I outgrown dyslexia? This incident which happened at the airport on the way home from Canada might help to answer that question.

I had been travelling for a month, skiing, relaxing, drinking beer and partying my head off. On my return trip to Australia I found myself in Hawaii with an eleven hour stop-over, feeling very 'stuffed' and wanting nothing more than a good sleep. Even though I was tired I intended to make the most of the stop over by hiring a car, getting some rays and seeing something of the countryside. It had always been a dream of mine to see Pipeline.

I realized that while I had been asleep on the plane other passengers had received their entry cards and had them filled in. This meant I had to leave the queue to go in search of one. This didn't take long but the crowd was gathering and the queue was lengthening while I struggled with the small print on the card.

Once I had filled it in with the information I thought they probably wanted I joined the queue again. Another few minutes of waiting and I presented the card to the customs official who looked at the card, then looked at me with some confusion and pointed out that I'd filled in the French side. He told me I'd have to go back and do another one. So I left the queue and went back to the counter where the cards were. This time I read the card more carefully. I filled in my name and then when it asked where I had come from I wrote Australia and similarly when asked where was I going naturally I wrote Australia. Feeling pleased with myself I once again very casually rejoined the queue, and waited my turn to step over the yellow line.

I handed my card and passport across the counter to the extra large Hawaiian customs officer. She took one look at it and told me somewhat disgustingly that I had filled it out incorrectly and I would have to do it again. Not wanting to go through the whole queueing process again I asked her if she would help me. She drew her large black pen out of her pocket, like she was drawing a sword, and proceeded to scrawl across my card. Maybe she had had a bad day, but it was about to get worse.

She asked me questions in short clipped sentences that did not attempt to disguise her annoyance at having to perform this additional duty. I was feeling pretty relaxed but becoming increasingly aware of her annoyance. In order to get back at me, it seemed, she sneered as she handed back my documents, and appearing to look straight through me, said, 'My four year old son could fill this card in better than you'.

Suddenly, I snapped. Perhaps it was my tiredness, I don't know but it was as if years of frustration, humiliation and battering surfaced inside me and I exploded. I stepped back in order to take a deep breath—somehow I knew what I was about to do and yet couldn't control it or hold it back. I can't remember exactly what I said but it was something to the effect that how dare you speak to me in this way when you don't know anything about me or what I have done. I was loud, abusive and determined to humiliate her as she and others before her had humiliated me. I had a great sense of power and invincibility and I was determined to make the most of it. Looking back I can see now that I was making an example of her to myself and was determined to defend my self esteem against someone I felt had no right to challenge it. In a perverse way I was enjoying it and aware that the whole customs area had stopped and was drawn to this spectacle. The customs officer retreated, belatedly aware that she had overstepped the mark—it was like a boxer retreating to the corner of the ring but I was holding her up determined to keep delivering the punches. I didn't care how she was feeling, I was too intent on avenging myself on the whole world of insensitive, uncaring, literate people.

The next thing I knew was that two other customs officers were approaching and telling me to 'settle down'. They attempted to manhandle me away from the scene but I shrugged them off and having expended my frustration I went with them, to an office near by. We were joined by the customs official and apologies were demanded. However so great was my sense of the justification of my actions (even though they weren't to know the real source of my anger) that I refused to apologize and challenged them to do their worst. Eventually they released me but not without some reluctance, and after a couple of hours had elapsed. I presented an image of defiance and determination but actually it was all a front—behind it all I was scared as hell and in my nervousness I left my passport behind which I only realized when I returned to the airport ready for my flight home.

I don't feel that my action matched the crime, but we must all be aware that what we see on the surface can be deceptive. Much the same as how a flat majestic river, with an excess of water can turn into a raging river. I don't see myself as an aggressive person, or someone that flies off the handle when something doesn't go my way. In fact I have never hit another person or been in a fight, although I did hit a teacher once, when I was in fourth or fifth grade. No matter what the situation I feel that violence is no solution. So I'm not saying that every individual you come across who treats you like a stupid moron or makes you feel socially incapable gives you the right to retaliate harshly.

I know that I was way out of line with the customs officer, but by absorbing her comments and frustration I would have only been increasing my self doubt and cementing it in even further than school did.

These days I don't get uptight like I did at the airport. Maturity has given me confidence rather than aggression, and I have learned new skills to combat the difficulties. Back at school one of my teachers wrote:

… copes well with his spoken English—but relies too heavily on this spoken form.

Today I use my verbal skills to my advantage. The phone book is not needed because you can use the operator, the street directory is hard to use so I just stop and ask until I get there; it may take longer but the end result is the same. Rather than write business letters I have face to face meetings or simply communicate by telephone. When I do have to write I can also get help with my spelling from my electronic dictionary.

So the problem is still there but it doesn't cause me nearly as much pressure as it did at school where I thought there would be no place in the community for someone like me. My dyslexia has faded into the background and only raises its ugly head in situations where there is no alternative. Sometimes I find myself in strange situations because of it and it makes life very interesting.

Even though I was categorized, graded and put into a box at school, I now realize that I didn't have to stay there forever. When I was travelling around in India I learned that over there you are born into a social class and that's where you must stay for the rest of your life. If you were born into the lower class your task was to wash clothes and your title was 'dobywaller' and 'dobywaller' you were for the rest of your life.

While it is important to realize your limitations it is just as important not to underestimate your own ability. We all have comfort levels which allow us to expand and grow to the boundaries of our limitations. But if the walls of your comfort level were broken down, there would be no limit to your ability to achieve or experience.

The only real limitation people have is themselves. Often we make our own boundaries. Instead of seeing myself as that negative picture of continual failure that I remember from my school days, I have chosen to recognize my learning difficulties and work on them as hard, or even harder, than the things I am good at. Some one like my self who has always been labelled as dyslexic, unable to cope with English, or dumb, must focus on those things that I can do. Self esteem, in regards to any personal problem we face, can sometimes be the difference between surviving and not. The day I started writing this story is the day I pushed myself beyond my own comfort zone. Even though books, teachers and words had always been my enemy the time had come to stop hiding and fighting and start believing that I could take one more look at my reading and writing problem.

Part 2

John—
A Case Study

John was born the third of four children and grew up with a brother who was 3 years older and two sisters, one 4 years older than he and the other 4 years younger. His birth was natural and without complication and his mother remembers him as a wonderful baby, so placid and contented. But while he was very undemanding, often needing to be woken for his feeds, his independent spirit was apparent from very early in his life. As soon as he was feeding from a bottle he insisted on holding it for himself. He was establishing a pattern of behaviour that has since characterised his whole life.

He lived a happy, carefree life in the years prior to beginning school. His family was kind and loving, with a comfortable home and the resources to be able to spend summer holidays at the seaside, enjoying each other's company. There were always plenty of children to play with and lots of activities for an energetic, adventurous little boy. In John's recollections of these early years can be found both his emerging strengths and the hints of possible difficulties to come.

One such hint can be found in his early crawling pattern. He preferred to crawl backwards! His mother describes how he would look to where he was going and then go towards it backwards. This may have been an indicator that his learning style would be different from most other children, or perhaps he was simply establishing early that he loved a physical challenge.

Nevertheless, researchers in the field of learning and learning difficulties have recognised that the way we learn to move as infants has far reaching implications for future learning behaviour. While all the developmental stages that the little child passes through are fascinating and vital, the crawling stage has been of particular interest to those who study patterns of learning. As a child learns to crawl, he or she is beginning to form those crucial connections between left and right sides of the body and hence is building communication between the left and right hemispheres of the brain. In addition, the crawling stage is providing the child with visual experience at a distance similar to that required for developing the future skills of reading and writing. By crawling, the child is creating important foundations upon which later learning is built. We don't know if the crawling style that John built for himself played a part in his later reading difficulties, but it was noticeably unorthodox.

When it came time for him to walk, he was confident and adventurous. Not for him the preliminary, hesitant steps taken while moving from one piece of furniture to the next. His mother remembers him pulling himself to his feet one day and he stood looking at her. Jokingly, she said, 'Come on Johnny, walk to Mummy', and to her amazement he did. A little unsteadily perhaps but with all the confidence and daring of the young man who would later ski downhill at a breakneck speed or launch himself over steep cliffs with only a rope and a few pegs for support. From a very early age, John trusted his body to take him where he wanted to go.

This willingness to fearlessly and joyfully accept a physical challenge, developed through his toddler years. He loved to ride his little trike as fast as it would go down the steep driveway at the side of his house, and head straight towards the garage doors. Then, just in time, he would skilfully turn the wheel and avert a disastrous collision. This dare-devil behaviour was repeated at kindergarten, where his teacher reported him giving her 'heart attacks' by swinging on the monkey bars and hanging upside down.

Later on he would try to keep up with his older brother and his friends, still on his little three-wheeler while they were riding on their bicycles. Even though they had a distinct advantage, he would pedal as hard as his little legs would go in an effort to catch up, often arriving home long after the others had returned from their ride, but never daunted by this or any other physical challenge.

In contrast to his physical prowess, John's language development was considerably delayed. Like many children, he developed a language of his own, and, while his mother could understand him, he would become very frustrated when others could not. He would resort to pointing gestures to get his message across and this situation did not improve greatly until he was 5 or 6 years old.

Research indicates that in a sample of people with dyslexic problems, 60 per cent had been late talkers. There is enough evidence to indicate that there is a strong possibility of future problems with reading and spelling if a child has any form of speech defect, or is still using immature grammatical structure at school commencement.[1] So, it would appear that language development can be a significant early warning sign that needs to be heeded and action taken to correct any problems as soon as possible.

However, it is not possible to foresee or avert all the events and experiences that have the potential to disrupt the equilibrium of the young, developing child. Sometimes episodes occur out of the blue and families simply cope as best they can. Just before John turned five, his favourite uncle was tragically killed. John's mother recalled, 'One is never the same after such a tragedy and even though you try to keep things normal, what effect this has on young children we will never know.' She felt that this event was especially significant in John's life because he and his uncle had been very close. It has been reported that the acquisition of the skills of reading and writing can be hindered or impaired by any social, emotional or physical problem that occurs, particularly prior to the age of seven, as it is in the infant grades that the foundations for literacy are laid.[2] This event in John's life might have compounded what was already a shaky start to school because of his speech delay.

Early signs of problems at school
John commenced school at the age of five years and one month and he was enrolled in a small private school catering to the infant grades. His parents

were not made aware of any problems with his learning during the first two years—this is the time when a dilemma can occur for parents and teachers. There is a need to remain flexible in regards to the expectations of what children should be achieving at certain age levels and so there is often an understandable reluctance to make unfavourable judgements about a child's early school progress. Yet, as already mentioned, it is precisely in these grades that significant fundamentals for literacy are acquired.

It was in Grade 2, perhaps with the prospect of transition to another school looming, that John's parents began to realise that his progress was not all that it should be. In order to provide him with a little extra help, a tutor was engaged for one hour per week. Unfortunately, this was not very successful as John resented having to sit indoors and do extra school work while the other neighbourhood children were outside playing. In addition, he had difficulty with the extra work he was being asked to do. Perhaps the tutor was trying to be helpful by providing work at a grade two level, but whatever the intention, John just couldn't do it. This only served to make him angry and frustrated.

Well meaning help, when it is not accompanied by a clear understanding of the learning process, can be counter productive. Much more is known today about the process of acquiring literacy than was known twenty years ago. Brian Cambourne, an Australian literacy/reading researcher, has identified five factors that may explain why students fail to acquire literacy:

1 faulty demonstration of the skills

2 students do not engage with the processes being offered
3 students' expectations of success are lowered
4 unhelpful feedback on attempts to read
5 all of the above.[3]

John may well have had 'all of the above' working against him, but quite clearly factor 2 was in operation—he was not really engaging with the processes offered, especially during the tutoring sessions. John still remembers being stuck inside while his friends were outside enjoying themselves and it is unlikely that this situation would have led to John's 'engagement' with the materials being offered, despite the best efforts of any tutor.

John's response, as an adult, to the issue of tutors, was to say that they should be organised to suit the child, rather than the parents and teachers—*Playtime is not the best time to be inside working on your English.* To be set apart from your friends in this way only served to make him feel 'like a retard'—not a useful emotion for a child wanting to be like his big brother. John reinforced this feeling on another occasion when he said that for him 'extra English was a negative ... I always felt that I was the different one in the family—we were all good at sport, we all had lots of friends ...' Drawing on his own experience, John suggests what at first glance may seem to be rather idealistic advice: *If a child is good at sport, why can't they learn while they are playing sport ... if they're good at music, why not let them learn while they're playing music?* There is wisdom in his suggestion, borne out by recent findings related to the way people learn. The crucial issue for John was acknowledgement of his learning strengths.

What John knows from his first hand experience, others have discovered through educational research—it is essential to acknowledge the learner's abilities and interests if we expect them to 'engage' with the learning process. While older learners may understand that the process they are engaged in will be to their benefit in the long run, it is very difficult for a small child to make that connection, and to make it with sufficient strength to overcome the immediate discomforts. From John's perspective, the little boy only understood that he couldn't do it, that there seemed to be no intrinsic rewards for him in trying to do it, and that he was being thwarted and prevented from doing the things that would make him feel good. In spite of the very best of intentions, during the entire process, what was being emphasised for him, were his learning weaknesses!

Patricia Vail, author of *Smart Kids With School Problems*, has argued strongly and persuasively for the acknowledgement, valuing and development of the considerable learning strengths which many dyslexics possess. She says:

Acknowledging the gifts and talents of dyslexic students, examining the curriculum we offer them, requires the next step of providing opportunity for them to stay in touch with their own strengths, and to show the world what they care about and what they can do.[4]

This of course has important implications for the building (or destruction) of self esteem—a crucial factor in effective learning. At the same time John's idea, based solidly upon his experiences as a 'reading disabled' student, substantiates the point that class teaching which has been inappropriate for the particular and unique needs of individual children, will result in them continuing to build and develop confusions and cover-up tactics. In John's case the evidence seems to suggest that his well meaning tutors ploughed on regardless, while he learned, and had reinforced, that he could not read; *he was learning to be learning disabled*.[5] He has said, 'It didn't matter how many times I tried to break a word up into different soundings, I couldn't do it.'

It is clear from this response, that John's early experiences of being 'helped' may not have had the desirable effects hoped for by his parents. On the contrary—what was intended to assist John, may have served to emphasise his difference and build barriers to the skills that the strategy was attempting to enhance. The issues at stake here are issues of timing—not only timing in terms of it being playtime outside, but more importantly, timing in relation to his need or purpose for learning. John summed this up when he wrote:

By allowing an individual to grow and develop the necessary tools to get through life can't be done in line with everyone else at the same age. It has taken me to the age of 25 to only just start to appreciate the need for the extra work that is needed to get me through life, and to progress with extra English.
And I have been doing extra English for as long as I can remember.

Primary School
At the beginning of his Grade 3 year, John moved from his small, private infant school to a much larger

Catholic boys' school. If he had experienced difficulties in kindergarten and infant school with the small pupil/teacher ratio, things were to become much worse for him at his new school. Because of the student numbers, John's mother recalled that everyone seemed to be taught the same, regardless of ability or personality. Whether John's behaviour actually became more disruptive at this school, or whether there was simply less tolerance for those who did not 'fit in', he nevertheless spent a great deal of time banished from the classroom. His mother remembers seeing him sitting outside the classroom whenever she would come to the school to help in the canteen.

In an effort to help him, his parents again arranged for extra tutoring and the school itself provided additional classes. His mother felt that all of this helped to some extent, but, in looking back, John was not so sure. He remembers the additional classes as being simply more of the same work that had been done in class already but 'only slower'—if the material contained little of interest to him the first time, it was even more boring when presented slowly in the repeated version. For a proud, energetic boy like John, there seemed to be little in these classes to engage his attention. As he pointed out in his stories, he did not consider himself to be a slow learner—he was a 'do-er'. Do-ers do not learn effectively by being made to sit still in desks for the duration of the school day. Then, working overtime, while plodding through material that is neither active nor enjoyable, makes the whole 'learning' process appear to be more like punishment. This was no one's fault in John's case—all concerned were doing the best they knew and maybe it did help a little.

Unfortunately it may also have helped to confirm in the child's mind that he was different, not smart, not like the other kids. This sort of awareness does not, of course, enhance a child's self esteem. Often this results in the child resorting to forms of behaviour which are deemed unacceptable to the school and the link between failure in the classroom and 'bad' behaviour can be seen in this excerpt from John's writing:

... being labelled as dyslexic at a young age is no easy thing to fight off in the playground: 'Here comes Brains ... ' or 'What mark did you get in the spelling test, Brains?' Putting me in a special class, labelled and life was not looking too pretty in those early days and it didn't get any easier.

John's way of dealing with this was to do what he was becoming very good at—being a class disturbance.

His mother, too, records this as a period of great frustration for John both at home and at school, and described him coming home from school, particularly in his grade 4 year 'very despondent, his head hanging on his chest'. Perhaps the thoughts he was able to articulate so well nearly 20 years later may help us to appreciate how he was feeling:

If for long enough you get told that you're not good at some things, regardless of your own personal strength, with time you will start to believe what is said. One's personal self picture is so important for growth and improvement otherwise all those negative thoughts will overwhelm you and with no effort your action and results will lead down the path of failure ... I felt in my earlier days that I knew the work, I even felt like I was quite good at it, but as time went by I seemed to fall further and further behind and before long labelled and put on the 'Extra English' shelf for life.

This sense of knowing the work, wanting work that matched his interest and intelligence, and yet being unable to effectively communicate that, was a source of great stress in his young life, so perhaps it should come as no shock that this manifested in the range of other 'symptoms' as well. He reported wetting the bed until he was ten or twelve, although his mother didn't think it went on for that long. He also remembered nightmares of never being able to keep up (shades of the little boy on the three wheeler bike), 'as if I was always fighting with life'. His sister would say that during the night she could hear him fighting with someone or something. He would grind his teeth, yell out loud and sleep walk. John feels that these behaviours were related to his problems at school.

In Grade 5 he was taken to the first of a series of experts for assessment and a program of planned assistance. The consultant was a speech therapist who had made a reputation for himself locally within the learning difficulties field. John's mother found comfort in his help as he did lots of tests and seemed to be able to isolate and explain where the problem was.

He established a program of learning skills to help John and one of John's former teachers from his infant school was employed to tutor him twice a week after school. The result was that although he tried hard, he was not able to get there quickly enough. His mother felt that this program too became a great trial for John, who was only too aware of the effort and sacrifices he was making for what seemed like very little result. Contributing to this was his reluctance to do the extra work in front of his brother and sister—once again his sense of not wanting to seem different may have been a significant barrier to his engagement with the learning process.

Yet in spite of his disruptive behaviour in class, John was not completely opposed to school; he wanted to succeed and be valued for what he could do rather than be constantly reminded of things he could not do—and these character traits are still very much a part of him. His mother wrote of his delight when, on her advice, the class teacher gave him 'a job', despite her initial reluctance because she said he was so naughty that he didn't deserve it. He was given the responsibility for cleaning the blackboard. His mother remembers him coming home with a big smile on his face and feeling so pleased with himself, and the result was that the complaints from school were considerably reduced for a long time. His mother saw this as an indication that, 'mothers aren't stupid and should be listened to and worked with instead of against as we found was often the case'.

However in spite of these improvements, by the end of Grade 6 it was clear that it would be in John's best interest for him to transfer to another school as his reputation was definitely working against him at the Catholic school.

Junior Secondary School
John's progression to a prestigious Grammar School, his mother knew, would not be easy for him because

his brother and sister, both of whom he looked up to, were at the school and she felt that as a very proud 12 year old his reading and spelling difficulties would be an enormous load to carry and work through. John remembers his first few weeks travelling on the bus out to the school, as being very traumatic and said that, although his parents didn't realise it, he would cry every day on the way to the bus.

One of the first difficulties he encountered was in finding his way about the large complex; he had difficulty finding his room and would get very confused, his mother wrote. John says that even now he experiences difficulty with directions and will say left when he means right and vice versa.

At the Grammar School, it appears that John's difficulties continued. He took piano lessons because his parent thought this might be 'a good thing', but, overwhelmed by all the new demands being made upon him, he would often forget to attend his lesson and so after 12 months this activity was dropped. Another 'extra' which was not making any worthwhile contribution to his school life was French, and during his second-form year his parents were called to a meeting with his House Master, English Master and French Master who reported that John had 'dug his toes in' and would not attend French. His mother reported that 'the penny dropped' when John asked how he could be expected to do French when he couldn't even do English. The solution at this time was for him to spend his French lessons in the library learning a French poem from a tape recorder because he was much better with the spoken than the written word. But one cannot help but conclude, that the principal consideration, from the school's point of view, was how to avoid having him wandering about the school during French class and it is ironic that it took John to point out why learning French was problematic for him. Fortunately he was heeded and it appears from his notes that at some stage an alternative to the French poem must have been organised because he wrote:

The only good extra English I had was when I didn't have to go to French because everyone else was going in different directions then, so I didn't feel like a retard.

His parents were pleased with the outcome because John was treated with respect and not made to feel inadequate.

In early secondary school, John was referred to another learning consultant. His mother took him to Melbourne on a series of visits and saw it as a positive step, as it helped her and John's dad to gain a little more insight into John's problems. They felt sure all these extra consultants helped. However, John was unimpressed with the notion of being taken to another expert to be evaluated. He does concede though, that Professor C's assessment of his academic future, as far as that school was concerned, was fairly accurate. John did have the impression though, that the professor was suggesting that he would be unable to continue with any academic work but should instead look for a trade or an apprenticeship. Without the actual report we cannot check on his wording and the implications that can be drawn from this, but there is no doubt that in John's mind the Professor had prescribed a limited future for him academically. It was a great source of satisfaction to John to be able, ultimately, to prove the professor wrong!

John's father's recollections of the visits to the professor are more positive:

As I remember, Professor C's theory was to develop John's strong school points. Make him happy and contented on positive things. Well, John developed these special skills—sport.

As indicated in his writing John feels very strongly about being excluded from discussions that relate to him and being kept ignorant of the processes in which he was involved. In an interview in which we discussed this point he indicated that he felt powerless in these encounters and he did not like it. It appears that the mysteriousness surrounding the tests he was given compounded the concern he had, and the feeling he was trying to keep at bay, about whether he was really stupid. He said:

… *they'd never tell you what you were meant to have been doing … and if they'd done this I would have known what he was trying to achieve and I would have been able to tell him instead of him doing all these tricks and making me work with blocks and then sitting down and writing these papers that you never saw.*

It is apparent from these comments that had he been shown a little more of the respect that his mother referred to earlier, and not made to feel inadequate, as these encounters certainly did, he may have mounted less resistance to the process. John comes back to the issue of respect on a number of occasions in terms of both the giving and receiving: 'If people treated me like a stupid moron, I would lose respect for them'.

John was fortunate that his parents were able to send him to a school that entitled him to spend his entire Year 9 at a campus of the school located in the mountains. While regular school work was an important factor, much time was devoted to outdoor activities emphasising fitness, self reliance and independence. Here John was in his element—a place where even the punishments were something to be exalted in; these generally involved having to get up early in the morning and run up and down the mountain—a task he loved. His mother recorded that even before year 9 he was developing into a good skier, surfboard rider, golfer and tennis player. With all of the outdoor activities available to him at the school he was able to add to his physical/sporting achievements.

John's school reports from Year 9 onwards are a valuable resource. Even though he categorised himself as a 'G SET retard', his reports from this year are very positive. The school explained the term 'G-Set' in an Explanatory Note to Accompany Term Reports—Sets are graded in ability ... students are assessed for these subjects within these Sets. The students' assessments should therefore be viewed in the context of the Set.

John's grades ranged from A through to C with the majority being B or B+. In third term he received an A in History, Mathematics, Physical Education, Geography and Science. Even acknowledging that these scores were assessed as part of the 'lowest stream', they were excellent for a boy who had such a history of struggling with his school work. The comments that accompanied these reports were also glowing with praise:

... high standard, positive attitude, continued to work hard, energetic, interested and most co-operative, keen and conscientious.

His third term English report is worth quoting in full:

John demonstrates his enjoyment of writing descriptively and vividly by making good use of similes and a varied vocabulary. He uses paragraphs correctly, varies his sentence beginnings and presents his ideas logically. His spelling and reading skills, although showing a marked improvement, are well below average. Grade: B

Such a positive and encouraging assessment acknowledges the difficulties without giving them undue prominence. His Phys Ed and hiking reports were also excellent, emphasising his enthusiasm, willingness to accept challenges and developing sense of responsibility. Then, the end of year unit report stated:

John has finished the year on a very strong note and seems set to make an excellent start to his time in senior school.

Finally, John had found a learning environment in which he could excel. In that environment, his physical skills were valued and developed and the benefits transferred to his other subject areas.

Senior Secondary School.
The contrast with John's reports just one term later could not be more marked. Apart from Phys Ed, for which he achieved a B grading, every other subject was rated E, even though attitude was at worst variable and at best good. Although the achievement Grade E officially meant 'having difficulties' for John it was a major disappointment and to him spelled FAILURE. The comments from his teachers lack the optimism and encouragement of the previous year:

Progress to the best of his ability

… concentration span is very limited

… does not appear to have much confidence in his own ability

The comparison between the end of Year 9 and the beginning Year 10 Science reports graphically illustrate his change.

Term 3 Year 9: *John's level of attainment has continued to be very good over the course of this term. Thus the year as a whole has been a grand success for him and he has given every indication that he enjoyed the course. His industry and application have been excellent and his study work habits should ensure a flying start to his time in senior school.*

Unfortunately they did not. The same teacher wrote just one term later in Year 10:

*Achievement E
Effort/Attitude—variable
Compared to his performance in this subject last year John has been through an extraordinary term. It has been dominated by huge fluctuations in mood and behaviour which has severely affected his output of work. I know he is capable of better attainment levels and look forward to seeing him return from holidays in a settled frame of mind.*

Again the teacher was to be disappointed. In Term 2, John's science report read:

*Achievement E
Effort/Attitude—not satisfactory
This has been a less successful term for John in that he has not applied himself as well and has again achieved low marks. He cannot concentrate for any length of time and is something of a hazard in the laboratory while experiments are being conducted. He has found chemistry very difficult to understand and I dare say next term's physics will cause further problems.*

His school work was clearly on a down hill slide and yet, through it all, his teachers reported that 'he has remained a cheerful personality who relates easily to other members of the set.'

In spite of overall effort and attitude results that were good or at least satisfactory, John's achievement grades were still in the D–E range. His Extra English reports referred to 'severe spelling difficulties' along with 'limited and ill constructed vocabulary'. He was chided for relying too heavily on his spoken English while acknowledging that he coped well with this.

Again, with the benefit of hindsight, it is possible to see that John may well have benefited from being encouraged to develop those skills with which he coped well, but it is apparent that the standards against which John was now being measured were no longer relative to his skill level but appear to be externally determined. He was to observe in his writing years later—it didn't matter how hard he tried or how much he improved, he would still get an E. In relation to this point he revealed one incident in which an English teacher said to him:

John you should not take your failure of English to heart. Some very famous people have gone through life with little or no written or reading skills. You have a great imagination and that is better than most English teachers, so keep trying and don't let those marks get you down.

In reply John said, 'If it's not such a big thing why didn't you give me a pass?' But the system he was now involved in, had no room for such flexibility. Against the criteria that were being used, he just didn't measure up. And the following year was no better. 'Well, the tussle continues', wrote the headmaster at the end of Term 1, 1982, in reference to the ongoing battles between John and the authorities in his school.

There is little doubt, from John's accounts, that at times his behaviour was more than just typical school boy pranks—there was hostility. This was aimed particularly towards teachers who he felt treated him like 'a moron', but also in many ways, towards a system which seemed bent on proving how inept he was. Clearly, this hostility served a 'self preserving function'. It provided a means of maintaining some semblance of himself in the face of evidence which seemed to indicate that he was 'the dumbest boy in the class', when he knew that he was not. In fact, he felt that he had more ideas that 'half the class put together'. Yet, while he seemed at times to take delight in making a nuisance of himself, he was still genuinely trying to cope with the work. His English teacher wrote most encouraging reports over the three terms of Year 11:

Term 1 *I am pleased with his determination to succeed—a commendable attitude that I hope he will sustain.*

Term 2 *... has worked well throughout the term, always being prepared to seek advice and guidance and trying hard to improve. One cannot ask for more.*

Term 3 *I am full of admiration for the commendable effort made by John to improve his written English. No one could have tried harder.*

No one could have tried harder—and yet, in spite of a clear acknowledgement of the *effort* being made, in Terms 1, 2 and 3 he was graded E; the official result sheet for the end of Year 11 gave E as 'below pass standard' and F 'well below pass standard'. This whole concept of failure in spite of great effort and improvement, is one which John finds inconceivable:

Imagine putting a whole year's work into something you loved, to be told that you had failed.

He was well able to prove himself on the sports field and, in fact, performed well enough in this to have earned his house colours a year early—not through skill in any one area but through his all round ability. However the 'colours' were not awarded because the housemaster claimed that his academic work was letting the house down and his house spirit was not adequate. So his strengths were being used to punish him and, even in sport, his writing difficulties were the means by which he was evaluated.

The culmination of this attempt at Year 11, was a letter to his parents from the housemaster, detailing what the school considered to be John's options. As a result of 'discussions' conducted at the school it was finally decided that rather than repeat the year, John would seek an alternative. John had no desire to give up, in spite of the struggle and the defeats. He knew that he wanted to work in the field of outdoor education and for that he would need a tertiary qualification.

He and his parents sought alternatives and to his immense joy, he was able to enrol in Year 12 at a government secondary school, even though in his eyes he 'cheated' to get in by not revealing that he had failed Year 11. His mother saw it 'as a chance for him to achieve the almost impossible academically, get Year 12 and go to Bendigo College.' She sympathised as he rode off on his bike to the other side of the city, wondering how this proud, handsome, enthusiastic, energetic, young man would manage to go through all the bluff to cover up for the fact that he could not read and spell very well.

His Year 12, in spite of some anticipated set backs largely related to his reading and writing problems, was a great success. He entered into the spirit of the school with enormous drive and vigour; he performed in the school play and participated in a variety of extra-curricular activities. In addition, he secured a voluntary job with a fitness centre which was part of his plan for getting into his outdoor education course.

John's English teacher best sums up John's approach to his Year 12, when she wrote eight years later, 'I will not forget his courage and will to succeed'. With some special consideration in terms of extended time to complete his exams and consideration in the marking, John was able to pass Year 12, including the examination for Physical Education—a pass in which was vital if he was to gain entry to his tertiary course. John accepted the need to pass this subject, in order to have any hope of getting in to the course he wanted, but he couldn't resist the comment, 'I felt you didn't need to spell *sport* or *teaching*, in order to do it'. He added, 'I know some P.E. teachers that are so fat they can't see their feet; that doesn't mean they can't teach someone else how to do push ups or gym.'

Tertiary Education.
John's results, along with a very successful interview, enabled him to be accepted into the outdoor education course upon which he had set his heart. Again, he had a great many hurdles to climb before this course would be satisfactorily completed. With assignments, he would usually have a friend correct his punctuation and spelling before handing in any work, or would send it home where it would be corrected (again only spelling, not the ideas), typed and sent back. But on one occasion, lack of time forced him to hand in work uncorrected and this

resulted in him being called to the Dean's office where he saw his work with red pen all over it. According to John, 'It looked like it had been to war. The lecturer had been so disgusted with my work, he had sent it to his Dean. The notes written all over it were not complimentary ...'

As a result of this he was threatened with expulsion, but fortunately he had an ally in another lecturer who supported his case. John had written to this lecturer after being accepted into the course, explaining the problems he had with reading and writing. However, he explained that he wanted no special privileges as a result of this but to be treated the same as everyone else. Nevertheless, both he and the lecturer realised that there are times when other strategies are warranted. When the lecturer entered the Dean's office John remembered, 'A quick chill came over me, for I knew that without his support I was history.' As a result of this support John was given a reprieve. Nevertheless it was not easy for him, and he spent his holidays redoing subjects in order to continue on the following year. Ironically, it was not as a result of his difficulties with reading but, because of an oversight in regard to a deadline, that John did not complete the course with his class. He graduated a year later, much to his disappointment.

Through these personal materials made available by John it has been possible to trace the developing frustration and distress which became a major feature of almost his entire school career. At the same time there is evidence of the 'fight back' strategies, which are common to many failing students and which enabled him to at least maintain some sense of control in a hostile environment. Other crucial factors in John's ultimate success were his own optimism and strong sense of purpose, along with an overall positive sense of himself. This was aided by his natural physical skills and the opportunities he had to develop these. Underlying all of these, was the love and support he could always count on from his family.

In summary, some key issues that have emerged from John's experience are:

1 That failure is cumulative;

2 That 'bad behaviours' may well be a healthy reaction to a self-threatening situation;

3 That to judge a person's learning ability, or their intelligence, on the basis of their ability to read and spell is to apply far too narrow a criterion;

4 That on the basis of early school experiences, learners may learn to become 'learning disabled'.

5 That learning success is possible if the teaching style or criteria for assessment are more flexible and creative.

Part 3   *How to Help*
_____

Brief Historical Background
The struggle to understand the nature of the particular difficulties associated with learning to read and write has been going on for at least one hundred years. Back in the 1890s, a Glasgow eye surgeon named James Hinshelwood, began reporting cases of what he termed 'congenital word blindness'. He drew attention to the problem in children who were otherwise healthy and intelligent. He was concerned that children experiencing such difficulties be given appropriate help otherwise he was afraid that 'they may be treated harshly as imbeciles or incorrigibles, and either neglected or punished for a defect for which they are in no way responsible'. Hinshelwood's fears were well founded and despite his concerns, many children suffered the pain and humiliation caused by years of struggling through schools which at best tried unsuccessfully to help them and, at worst, blamed and punished them for their difficul-

ties. As a result, many such children left school at the first opportunity and remained convinced throughout their lives that they were dumb and would never amount to much.

A quarter of a century later Samuel T. Orton, an American neurologist, recognised the condition described by Hinshelwood, in a young patient of his own. Orton came to believe that difficulties with learning to read and write were the result of faulty brain functioning stemming from the failure of one brain hemisphere to establish dominance over the other. He used the term 'strephosymbolia' in preference to 'word blindness'. Orton founded a society that continues to conduct research and develop techniques and strategies to help people learn to read and write more successfully. The Orton Dyslexia Society, as it is now known, is active in a number of countries and conducts conferences, seminars and workshops to train people in the teaching methods which have their origins in the work of Dr Orton.

In the late 1970s another American, a researcher and remedial educator, Dr Paul Dennison, developed a systematic program of movement based activities designed to balance the energy flow and communication between the two hemispheres of the brain in order to facilitate ease of learning. Dr Dennison discovered that people are not so much learning disabled as learning blocked. This may be the result of a number of factors ranging from insufficient movement in infancy to stressful learning experiences at any stage of the learner's life. Dr Dennison's work is called Educational Kinesiology and his basic program of movement activities is known as Brain Gym. The Educational Kinesiology Foundation, which he established, also conducts research and international seminars and training programs in order to pass on his discoveries.

Over the past century a great deal of research, both formal and informal, has been undertaken in countries all around the world in an effort to better understand and find more effective ways of dealing with dyslexia. Books have been written and vast numbers of reports and papers have been compiled; medications have been introduced and various medical theories advanced; new methods of teaching have been tried, and old methods revived and refined and yet the problem continues to exist. Children continue to struggle through school, never quite measuring up and being left with the sense that they are not as smart as other kids, or worse still, that there is something wrong with them which makes them incapable of learning effectively.

This feeling has been reflected over the years in the variety of labels that have been devised in an attempt to more adequately define the problem. These have included 'minimal brain dysfunction', 'reading retardation', 'specific reading disability', 'learning disability', and 'specific learning disability'. Each label has been superseded by another, as the search continued. Labels, of themselves, contribute little towards overcoming the difficulties of trying to learn to read and write, but a non-offensive label (and there is little doubt that John would have found all of the above offensive in the extreme) can offer some comfort to people struggling to understand difficulties for which there is no adequate explanation.

Being able to label their difficulties with a clinical term removes from people the burden of being 'stupid'. 'Dyslexia' serves this purpose as well as any other term and better than most. The British actress

Susan Hampshire, who has written two books about her experiences of dyslexia, says that as a child she heard terms like 'mental' and 'retarded' being used about her and she wondered why. Eventually the term 'word blindness' was used and it was a relief to her to find that her difficulties had a name.[1] While 'dyslexia' is more likely to be the label used today, the effect is usually the same. Relief, that those difficulties have a name.

What are the symptoms of Dyslexia?
First of all, 'symptoms' suggests that it is a medical condition, and we do not know that this is so. But given that, this question usually means that people want to know whether their child is just a little behind in their reading and writing or if there is something really wrong.

Sometimes you will find lists of difficulties containing items like the following:

- Difficulty in distinguishing left from right
- Clumsiness
- Disorganised
- Reverses letters
- Leaves out words or substitutes words when reading
- Awkward hand writing
- Spelling difficulties, often with no obvious pattern to the mistakes.

These are just a few and the list could go on and on, but the main issue would seem to be that the learner has a specific difficulty with reading and writing skills, but may be excellent in other areas. This results in them functioning at a level considerably lower than that which would be expected for their age and intellectual ability.

Apart from the relief factor mentioned above, the only real advantage in being able to identify Dyslexia precisely, would be if there were a wonderful program or treatment which would get rid of it. There are many things which may help, but there is no one cure, strategy or treatment that will work for everyone because there is no one condition called Dyslexia. Every person struggling with difficulties associated with reading and writing, is experiencing their own unique set of circumstances and knowing how to help them requires a very open mind and a wide range of helping strategies.

Identifying Learning Styles
Good teachers have always endeavoured to cater to individual differences within the classroom. This may have involved recognising that some children need more time than others, that concentration spans vary considerably or that different levels of work need to be provided during a lesson. What we are now beginning to understand is that an important key to understanding individual differences and thus a key to helping people learn more effectively, lies in finding out HOW they learn.

John is able to explain what works for him in his learning and can describe his learning strengths. In his own words, he is a 'do-er'. In saying this he is actually drawing attention to the fact that learning occurs most effectively for him when he is physically involved in the process.

... to me learning is like life. I must experience, feel and be a part of it. To gain the true meaning

of something I need to see it—like digging a hole. At the end of the day you can see what you have done ... but it must also have meaning and purpose for me to learn and I must feel that I am going to gain something at the end of it. Enjoyment during the process is just as important as the end result.

Yet to read a book about Shakespeare off that shelf means nothing to me and I can't relate to it. I like to be a part of it. And I can't see myself standing at the bottom of the window asking Juliet for sex. I would have climbed the tower!

We need to pay much more attention to the things which people are able to learn successfully, if we are to help them with the things which don't come so easily. This is why my opening question to John, on our first meeting, was 'How do you learn?' followed by 'Tell me about something which you have learned really successfully and joyfully'. That of course led to the discussion of skiing. While there might seem to be a world of difference between learning to ski and learning to read, I don't believe there is. As a child, John taught himself to ski by being left to his own devices and working it out for himself. He refused teachers and classes, preferring to find his own way of doing it.

John described to me the feelings and sensations involved in skiing: how he learned to recognise the feel of the snow beneath him and how this feeling could be translated through his feet, legs and whole body into an understanding of what it was like to ski. It sounded very much like reading, only he was reading his environment with his whole body.

Learning and Intelligences

This ability to be very sensitive to one's body and to read its messages effectively is essential for success in many fields of sport, gymnastics, dancing or even playing a musical instrument. It is, according to respected psychologist, Howard Gardner, one of the seven 'intelligences'. Gardner calls it 'Kinesthetic' or 'Bodily Intelligence'. He has identified that humans have the capacity to develop at least seven intelligences:

1 Linguistic   (to do with language)
2 Spatial   (relating to pictures, patterns, design, direction)
3 Mathematical/Logical
4 Musical
5 Bodily/Kinesthetic   (physical skills)
6 Interpersonal   (ability to relate to others)
7 Intrapersonal   (knowledge and understanding of self)[2]

Unfortunately, only two, Linguistic and Mathematical/logical are given 'high status' recognition as signs of intelligence in our society. The others tend to be regarded as extras. However, as Patricia Vail points out, it is these 'extras' 'which nourish the mind, body and soul of our society. These are precisely the intelligences many dyslexics have ...'[3] This evaluation might have been written specifically with John in mind. He is never happier than when engaged in activities involving particularly the Bodily/Kinesthetic, Spatial or Interpersonal skills, which he has in abundance. It was this strength, and his preference for learning in this mode, that his brother's friend was able to tap into when helping him to study for his final exam in High School. John once remarked that if as much time and effort had been expended in developing his sporting skill, as was used in trying to build his reading and writing, he'd have been an Olympic athlete by now. Wishful thinking perhaps, but maybe a more realistic assessment of his learning strengths than his schools acknowledged.

Learning Styles and Learning Strengths
By appreciating the diverse ways in which human intelligence is manifested we can begin to understand more about how to work with people's own learning strengths. It is only when we learn to acknowledge the valuable part that each of the intelligences plays in enriching all lives that an individual's true potential will be recognised and cultivated.

It would be silly to attempt to deny the importance of linguistic and mathematical/logical skills. They are essential for many of the most important areas of our lives, especially schooling and employment. However we do need to give considerable thought to finding the best ways of helping those, who like John, find themselves having difficulties mastering certain skills. John felt that much of the effort put into 'helping' him was wasted. It might help us understand John's reaction a little better if we were to consider two alternative areas of learning difficulty and what might be done to help.

What happens if a student is not succeeding musically? Is he or she categorised as 'dysmusical'? Is the lack of musical interest or talent seen as evidence of a generalised lack of ability or intelligence? Will the student be expected to take remedial music classes in their own time? Are they regularly expected to stand in front of the class and sing, when clearly this is not something they are ready to do? Are they made to produce their physical education or science reports in musical form and then graded accordingly? Can you imagine what their attitude to music, and probably school in general, would be if this were the case?

Let's use another analogy, this time from the area of kinesthetic/bodily intelligence. What happens if a small child at school is unable to catch a ball or kick a football as well as might be expected for their age? How would that child be helped? Firstly, the teacher might try to ascertain whether the inadequacy was simply due to insufficient opportunities to practise the skills well, or if there was an underlying visual or coordination problem for which more specialised activities or intervention were required. Provided vision was not a problem, the teacher would probably work on the skills with lots of games and fun activities that would enable the child to develop the techniques that were lacking. Being a 'butter fingers' can almost be as bad for a child as being dyslexic, especially in a society that places such high store by sporting achievements. So it is most important that the child's sporting self esteem not be damaged in the process of helping, because that negative self opinion can be a powerful block to any further attempts at effective helping. If the child were to be sent outside to practise catching balls that were thrown too high, too low, or too wide, until his or her arms ached, while all the other children were playing inside in a warm house, talking, laughing and enjoying themselves, no doubt the child would feel rather like John with his after school tutor. The child might feel excluded, different, inept, tired and possibly frustrated or angry—and none of these emotions are renowned for their ability to foster learning.

It is only when these 'helping' strategies are seen in the context of the other intelligences that it is possible to fully appreciate why they sometimes do not work as well as hoped. Tutors and parents do not set out to upset children and waste their time, but in their eagerness to do something, the end gets lost in the means. Learning occurs most successfully when there is a desire to learn, when the learner is encouraged, when they are able to see and feel success and when they are gaining enjoyment, or another equally positive benefit from the activity.

Visual, Auditory and Kinesthetic Learning
While Dr Gardner's list of intelligences provides one framework for understanding differences in individual learners, another way is through determining the order in which people/learners process information. This system uses the abbreviations V.A.K. to describe Visual, Auditory and Kinesthetic modes of processing. As learners, everybody accesses all three modes, but it would appear that we differ in the *order* in which we use them.

People who have a preference for processing information Visually like to be able to see what they are learning about. For them demonstrations, pictures, videos, diagrams and writing are all very important to their understanding. To deliver a lesson or lecture with no visual assistance would not be an effective way to communicate with such learners. They may communicate their understanding with expressions like—'I see', 'I get the picture' or 'That looks right' or alternatively, 'It doesn't look right', or 'I can't see what you mean'.

Those who have a preference for Auditory processing of information will gain a lot from the spoken word and may be able to concentrate for long periods while listening. They may say 'That sounds right' or 'That rings a bell with me', when acknowledging their understanding or use other expressions that relate to sounds and hearing.

For the other major category, the Kinesthetic learner, the preferred method of learning is to 'do'. To be involved, trying out, experimenting and getting the feel for what is being learned is essential for a thorough understanding. Such a learner might use the expressions like, 'I get it' or 'It feels right'.

Again, good teachers have always recognised the importance of presenting information in as many different ways as possible so that the diverse preferences within the classroom can be catered to. However, it has been through the work of Neuro-linguistic Programming theorists like Richard Bandler, John Grinder and Michael Grinder that this understanding has been thoroughly developed into a highly refined method of communication which can have far reaching applications for teaching and learning. They have recognised that while we use all three modes of processing to some extent, the order in which we use them can significantly affect our ability to make sense of the information with which we are being presented. Thus we find V.A.K. learners who need to see what is to be learned, then hearing about it will make more sense and finally they will try and do it for themselves. The K.V.A. learner on the other hand, wants to have a go first, then he or she can see what it looks like and after that an explanation will make more sense. Some learners (A.V.K.) prefer to hear something explained, then see a picture or diagram, before attempting to apply the information. These combinations of modalities, as they are called, will differ from one person to another.

In John's case, it would seem that his sense of touch, feel and general body awareness—his kinesthetic learning mode, is of major significance for him. His visual mode is the next preferred, as he is able to make good use of this once he has experienced something. The auditory mode would be last on his list. For John, as for many other learners, theory is most effectively built on a basis of practical/kinesthetic experience. There is nothing wrong with this—it is a very effective way of learning—once the pattern has been recognised and the learner's needs are addressed by the teaching style used.

Each style or combination of processing mode has it own characteristics. Ask a visual learner to do or make something before they have a clear *picture* of what is expected, you are likely to get a delayed or less than satisfactory response. Visual learners can often be identified as the ones who want to show you what they can do—*look at me, see what I have made* or *I want to see what you are doing*. This is quite different from the kinesthetics—*can I have a go? Let me do it. I want to try it.* They like to be involved. While they may make mistakes initially because 'You didn't listen to what I told you' or 'You didn't watch what I was showing you', nevertheless, they learn from their mistakes and, provided they are not discouraged from having another go, they will keep trying until they get it right.

Having an understanding of the preferred or

dominant mode of learning, as well as the order of access of the main senses for learning, are important factors in whether or not we will be successful learners. To be talked at, told, instructed, lectured, explained to will be likely to produce the 'deaf ear' response from someone whose least preferred mode of processing information is auditory.

For those who want to help children or adults become more proficient learners, the main thing to be aware of is that the one we are seeking to help may process information differently from the way we do. All three 'modalities' are important and someone is not 'smarter' just because they learn effectively by listening (although they may fit into the school/work system better), nor is someone less 'smart' if they do not respond well to verbal instructions. We need to maintain awareness of the three channels of communication so that if what we are doing is not working, we can try another approach. As John has pointed out, 'more of the same, only slower' is not very successful.

This awareness of learning styles was not well known when John was young. But looking back on his stories the signs of Kinesthetic Intelligence were there. As soon as he could walk his mother said 'He was busy, busy, busy, into everything.' The episodes with the small trike indicate a little fellow fearlessly exploring the limits of speed, balance, and body control. He could turn his trike at the very last moment, while hurtling at great speed towards the garage doors. He was not interested in sitting still and listening to stories or watching other people *doing things*, he wanted to be doing himself. His description of 'skiing in whiteout' may be reckless, perhaps even foolhardy, but for John, his confidence in his body's ability to read the environment, is supreme.

With the benefit of hindsight, we have to consider the effect of putting John into a desk, telling him to sit still and expecting him to learn primarily by listening. Clearly it did not work well for him, and in the process caused considerable harm to his confidence in himself as a learner. The idea of locating the cause of learning difficulties with the *educational experience,* rather than with the learner, is one which now enjoys wide support. The notion of failure in the teaching, rather than in the learning process, cannot be ruled out. Sadly, but fortunately, he had to wait till he was an adult to know that his form of learning is as valid as anyone else's—and as effective.

How does a 'do-er' learn to read and write?
We know that there are lots of 'do-ers' out there and no doubt a few of them will be experiencing problems with their school work. So how does a 'do-er' learn to read and write? The possibilities are limited only by the imagination of the people involved—but there do seem to be some key elements that will help.

1 Recognise and value the preferred learning style. This will mean that the learner will not be exposed to the idea that the way they learn is wrong. They will be continually affirmed that they are okay.

2 Recognise the importance of movement for learning. For too long there has been the view that kids who jiggle and get fidgety have short concentration spans. What if this were changed to an awareness that their concentration is linked to movement—when they are denied movement they lose their concentration and 'switch off'.

3 Think laterally—if kinesthetic learners switch off by being made to sit still for long periods of time, why not try standing desks for example, as an alternative in the classroom. This way they can stand and move in their own space.

4 Noticing when the *time* is right for learning may be crucial; this means being aware of the child's more likely 'switched on' and 'switched off' times and capitalising on these—certainly the end of the day, when everyone else is playing, will often not be a good time for the increased concentration needed for a tutoring session in reading.

5 Have as wide a range of instruction methods and materials as possible, with a heavy emphasis on active learning. There are books available which can help with suggestions here. Capitalise on the interests of the learner. Sometimes, books which appear too advanced will actually seem easier if the interest is there.

6 Keep the interest level high and respect the child's intelligence. As John said, there is nothing more boring than being made to do the same deadly dull work again and again at a slower rate. As he pointed out he does not learn *slowly*, he learns *by doing*.

This insight into John's learning gives us many clues about how to go about valuing the contribution and talents of any people who are having difficulties with reading and writing. Not all such people are 'doers'; they may have strong visual skills but are having trouble hearing the differences in letter sounds; or they may have excellent auditory discrimination skills but be unable to 'see' that 'b' is different from 'd'.

Nevertheless, whatever the source of their difficulties, they may have a number of strengths in common. Patricia Vail[5] identified ten traits which she believes characterise many intelligent students unable to read or write successfully. They are:

1 Rapid grasp of concepts—knowing the answer but having no idea of how you got it. John mentions that often he felt like he knew all the answers but he couldn't explain.

2 Awareness of patterns—this was identified as an ability to understand patterns in nature for example. This equates with John's ability to interact so effectively with the environment through sport, rock climbing and even his ease in interpreting a contour map.

3 Energy—this refers to high intellectual energy and can be seen in an ability to pursue an idea and see a project through to its conclusion. John's energy in pursuing the idea of this book, is a principal example of this.

4 Curiosity—this is part of the pursuit of knowledge and understanding or experiencing that is a feature of these high energy people.

5 Concentration—this may be accompanied by a poor sense of time, so that the concentration does not manifest itself in line with school subjects or school schedules but is apparent when the issue or activity is of relevance to the learner.

6 Exceptional Memory—once again while this may not appear to be the case because of the difficulties associated with remembering spelling rules or mathematical tables, it may take the form of experiential or emotional memory. John's reference to being able to describe in details all about the places he has visited in his travels yet be unable to remember the specific names of countries fits with this.

7 Empathy—this is the ability to sense and feel how another person is feeling and is a form of intuition.

8 Vulnerability—this means the emotional vulnerability of the person to the pain that is experienced as a result of the learning problem. We can see this in John's stories of his restless sleep, tears on the way to school and even hiding in the toilets to avoid having to read aloud.

9 Heightened perceptions—this included for John an ability to sense when someone was in sympathy with him and when they were against him.

Some of John's most successful learning experiences have occurred in learning situations where he perceived the teacher was sympathetic to his difficulties. On the other hand, he is able to make very rapid assessments of people who are not genuine or who are negative.

10 Divergent thinkers—these people are not deterred in any way by tackling a problem which might seem to others to be impossible or at best too difficult. There is plenty of evidence of this trait in John.

Is there a right or wrong way to help?
It is vital that if children are to be given extra tutoring, that it be useful and helpful. The program must be one that will produce a result for that child and not

one that will reinforce failure. Because John did not form a sound basis for literacy in his junior primary years, in spite of extra tuition, his problems were compounded in later primary school and aggravated by large class sizes and an impersonal system unable to deal with one child's specific problems.

Children, finding themselves in John's situation, will generally react along a continuum. At one extreme, we can expect some may be likely to withdraw, becoming very quiet and compliant, wanting above all not to draw attention to themselves and their problems. Or like John, they may go the other way, lashing out in frustration and anger and becoming skilled in disruption and bad behaviour. Neither reaction will be very helpful in regard to learning, but both need to be recognised as ways of reacting to what is an extremely stressful, frustrating and even humiliating situation. We only need to imagine how we would react to the situation of having to work at something we could not master, for years on end, to be subjected to daily reminders of our failure, to begin to appreciate the degree of stress involved.

Unfortunately once the self protective behaviour takes over (whether it be withdrawal or disruption) the individual is no longer in effective learning mode. Hopefully this defensive, unproductive state can be broken by building self esteem through recognising and acknowledging strengths, skills and talents, building on these and using them as a basis for literacy learning.

It is often surprising how easy it is to create a positive, self esteem building situation. Remember John's delight and pride when he was given the job of cleaning the blackboard. Praise for jobs well done (and not necessarily jobs associated only with school or school work) and the allocation of small positions of responsibility, can work wonders.

On the other hand, in a situation where one child is at a disadvantage compared with others in the family, the potential for damaged self esteem is considerable. Being put down, even unintentionally, with comments like, *We never had that problem with your sister* or *Why can't you do as well as your big brother?* only reinforces a sense of failure and disappointment. Even if no one openly compares their performances unfavourably, they know that they are different. This makes it all the more important that they have their area(s) of expertise developed whatever it is, and that this is acknowledged and valued.

Practical Ideas To Help With Reading And Writing

The following suggestions may assist you to more effectively help a student/learner:

1 Be aware that the way you learn things may not necessarily be the way your child or student learns. Do notice the things they are good at and see what ideas you can pick up from this to help them with their reading and writing. For example, if they enjoy drawing, introduce plenty of colour and design features into their writing tasks; if they like music, use tunes and rhythm to get the information across. Notice what works and do it.

As far as possible organise the experience to fit with the child, rather than trying to get the child to fit into a particular method or time of day or length of session.

Things to look for might include:

(i) Concentration span—of course the concentration span for something they are interested in will be vastly different from something that holds no interest. So notice what is a reasonable length of time to expect them to concentrate on reading or spelling. Break sessions up into short, regular periods of time—10 minutes, six times per week may be far more effective for some learners than one hour weekly.

Such an arrangement may not only cater more effectively to the child's concentration span, but will also give the much needed reinforcement for their memory. It has been shown that recall of newly learned material is significantly improved if that material is reviewed within ten minutes of learning, then within 24 hours, again within one week and then periodically after that.

(ii) Do they seem to learn well, more by doing, watching or listening? Adapt your helping strategies to *their* learning preference.

(iii) How do they look when they are relaxed and enjoying what they are doing? Note their posture and facial expression. It is important to recognise the signs of boredom and frustration because these indicate you are probably wasting your time trying to help at this time.

(iv) What subjects are they interested in or, better still, engrossed in? This information will give you hints about the choice of reading material. Even if their choice of subject may not appear to you to be very worthwhile, remember the primary purpose of the exercise—if you want to help this child to read, it may not be contributing to the goal to have him or her read material which you think is suitable, but the child regards as boring or irrelevant.

2 Be aware that some of the mental processes involved in reading 'out loud' are different from the ones required for silent reading and comprehension. Therefore it is possible that a child who stumbles and reacts hesitatingly when asked to read aloud, may actually be able to understand what they are reading about, if the pressure to 'perform' is removed.

Games associated with questions and answers about the material being read will soon establish, in a relaxed way, whether it has been understood. Don't forget too, that it can be just as instructive to have the child think up a question about the piece for you to answer, and this again takes the pressure off them to always be the ones to have to find the answers.

3 Looking at the pictures and using whatever clues are available to find out what the story is about is NOT cheating. This is especially important for young readers, because we need to be helping and encouraging them to see themselves as successful readers and this means broadening our ideas about what constitutes reading.

The greatest disservice we can do to young readers is to build into them a sense of failure or of being 'wrong'. This doesn't mean we have to praise everything they do—be selective or the praise will lose its value, but be ready and willing to support them in all their efforts to extract meaning from their books.

4 When trying to spell it can be encouraging to the learner to be shown that only part of their spelling of a word is wrong. The all or nothing approach means that when one letter is wrong the whole word is called 'wrong'. But if there is one letter missing or they got a couple of letters in the wrong place, let them know they got at least part of the word right, rather than leaving them to think they have to re-learn the entire word.

This might seem a minor consideration but I have noticed the looks of disappointment on students' faces when they are told their word is wrong and how different they look when told—this word is 90 per cent right, or almost all right—'See, you've got all of these letters correct, there's only this one we need to concentrate on'.

5 Help the visual memory. Make use of colour and design to help difficult words appear more interesting and memorable. This establishes a visual image and aids recall. You can do this by:

(i) Writing each syllable in a different colour;

(ii) Highlighting the silent letter with colour or by making it bigger, or by turning it into a picture.

eg. S C H O O L   S C 🏠 O O L

(iii) Visualise the word in a context. For example, to help remember the 'au' in restaurant, a student visualised a restaurant in a forest of Autumn leaves. This helped to provide a link between a learned word and a yet-to-be learned word.

Researchers in Neurolinguistic Programming, studying human communication processes, have noticed that people turn their eyes upward when trying to remember something visually. For right handed people this usually involves looking up to the left and for left handers it might be up to the right—but either way it is up. So it may help to write the words being learned onto cards in colour and then hold them so that the eyes turn up to see them. This will assist the learner with recall as he or she will automatically look up when trying to remember and therefore may have more immediate access to the word stored in the visual memory.

If using this system, the following process may serve as a guide:

(i) Write the word clearly and in colour on to a piece of card.

(ii) Hold it so the learner's eyes turn up and to the left (or right if this seems appropriate) in order to see it.

(iii) When they have had a good look, ask them to close their eyes and ask questions like:

What colours were in the word?
How many letters were in green?
What was the first/last colour?
What colour was the big letter?

These questions are there to check whether they are beginning to form a visual picture of the word. Only when questions like those above can be answered successfully, do you move on to others that test the memory for the actual word. And whenever memory falters let them have another look—the whole purpose is to build a strong visual picture and keep it fun—keep the pressure OFF.

A good way to really check whether the visual picture is there is to ask them to tell you the letters they can see—*backwards*. This means they need to rely entirely on their picture and they won't be trying to sound it out at the same time. They will be amazed that they can do it. To make sure the image doesn't simply disappear in a day or so, it will be necessary for them to practise picturing it regularly but this can be done in the middle of drying the dishes or walking to school—it's just checking to see if it is still there visually, but in the checking they will be strengthening the image.

The more they are able to then incorporate the words into their reading and writing the more they will be reinforcing their memory for that word. Another message here is that desperately learning ten words for the spelling test at the end of the week will only be useful if the words being learned are likely to be used in the near future after the test—otherwise, as many children will tell you, 'I learned them for the test and now I've forgotten them'.

6 Make use of auditory memory by adding rhythm and rhyme to what is being learned. Singing spelling patterns might seem a bit silly, but the brain enjoys a bit of silliness and nonsense and certainly takes more notice—the rhyme will have even more impact if you can attach a visual picture to it. Putting similar words into funny sentences and saying them out loud is another auditory strategy, but to ensure the spelling of the words is also incorporated, once again a visual component is needed.

7 Investigate the use of music—there is a way of teaching and learning which recognises that music can have a significant effect on helping people to remember what they have learned. Because music can help to regulate the rhythms of your body including the waves of electromagnetic energy in your brain, having music playing while you or your child is learning can help to ensure that all of the brain is engaged in the process.

Considerable research has been carried out regarding the significance of music to learning. The method known as *Suggestopedia*, or more commonly Accelerative Learning, acknowledges music as an important factor in helping the brain to work in harmony with reduced stress. While there is not space here to go into detail—it must be said that not all forms of music are suitable either. Music with words attached is less appropriate because it encourages the verbal left brain to hone in on the words; similarly, music with a steady thump, thump beat is likely to encourage more left brain sequential involvement than a harmonious whole brain approach.

The type of music recommended in Accelerative Learning sessions is Baroque music, particularly that with a 'largo' beat. But I would not suggest that anyone should suddenly introduce this into a student's study environment. For some, particularly those who 'hate classical music', the stress of listening to it would be quite counterproductive to effective study.

Notice whether music seems to help, and trial different sorts of music in order to find the most appropriate.

8 Be aware of the 'suggestions' that you are making regarding the work to be done. Are you building an expectation of success by the things you are saying, or are you reinforcing a sense of failure? Statements which remind the learner of their experiences of success help to set them up for further success. When you say, 'You got most of your words right last night, wasn't that good!' you reinforce their ability to achieve. If you are finding it a bit hard to think of something positive to say about their spelling or reading, then you need to look carefully at the work they are doing. Is it too difficult? It may be necessary to back-track until you can find something they can do successfully and then build up from there. They need to know what it feels like to experience success with reading and writing otherwise they continue to set themselves up for failure and unconsciously develop blocks to learning. And to do this, they might first need to focus on the way success feels in a totally unrelated environment.

How important is Spelling?
Quite clearly in many people's minds it is extremely important; if you can't spell you must be a bit of a dunce. It seems to me that what is infinitely more important is that firstly the learner has the *confidence* to write and secondly he or she has the *ideas* to express.

Writing can be a wonderful tool for self-discovery as well as a means of communication and recording information. By writing, it is possible to discover ideas that you didn't know you had; writing will encourage clarification, expansion and further discovery. This has certainly been John's experience and that of many other students. The pity is that too many people equate writing with spelling and because they know their spelling is bad, or faulty, they don't write.

There is no doubt that poor spellers today, who have access to a word processor with a 'spell check' facility have a great advantage over their fellow sufferers of a few years ago, whose only strategy was to 'Go and look it up in the dictionary'—very difficult, when you don't know how to spell it in the first place. Every effort needs to be made to learn how to spell correctly, and the earlier the better, because this will save time and make writing easier and more pleasurable. When writing is for a wider or more critical audience, it must be correct. With the availability of computers and word processors the tools are now accessible for all writers to turn out a perfect finished product. Students today are much more familiar with the whole concept of process writing and they no longer expect that their first draft will be their final product.

'Spell check' on the word processor will never replace the learned ability any more than the calculator will replace knowing your times tables—in both instances it is far quicker to do it by brain than by finger or micro chip. But as a checking device or as a means of learning to become a better speller, or as a back-up when spelling is an insurmountable obstacle to writing, it is a valuable tool to be used.

Is 'sounding out' the right way to tackle unfamiliar words?

There is a great deal of disagreement about the practice of 'sounding out' or 'phonics'. Some people have written books about how it is the only way to learn the basics of English. Other people will argue that it is useless as a method of teaching reading and writing skills and will only make matters worse. It is a battle that has been raging for many years, and promises to be around for many more. Whether one is arguing from one extreme or the other, or from a position somewhere in between, there is usually a good deal of research to back up disparate points of view; in other words there are strong arguments on all sides.

There is little doubt that some learners will be helped considerably by being given intensive instruction in phonics, by learning the sounds and sound combinations of the language, and by learning how to link these together to make words. But keep in mind that this method does not work well for everyone. John's experience bears this out. Be watchful and respect the learner's learning style. If the method is producing results, and the learner is comfortable with it, then it is a good method. But if it is not working, change it.

Proper instruction in phonics is a complex task and requires an extensive program (the Orton-Gillingham method, for example). Phonics improperly or incompletely taught, can be a source of confusion for the learner because of the many English words that do not lend themselves to a simple phonic approach.

Here is a compromise: If the word can be sounded out and the meaning gained then by all means use this method. Words like A-N-D or D-O-G or T-R-I-P or even D-E-N-T-I-S-T and other longer words lend themselves very well to being sounded out. However what happens when you try to sound out basic words like C-O-U-L-D and S-H-O-U-L-D? What about M-O-U-L-D or T-H-O-U-G-H-T or B-E-C-A-U-S-E? And then there are even longer words which require the learner to remember all the sounds in order to put them together into a word.

Another complication here is that some people simply have great difficulty putting isolated sounds together. It just makes no sense to them at all. So whether or not phonics or 'sounding out' is a good method depends firstly upon the words and secondly upon whether the strategy works for the person actually doing it.

An alternative to breaking words up into individual sounds is to learn about syllables and how to break words up this way. This must be accompanied by learning how sounds like 'sh' and 'ch' and 'th' go together to make single sounds. Letter combinations like *ow* as in 'cow' need to be contrasted with *ow* as in 'show'. Sounding out will not help a student to know that *ough* in 'bough' is different from *ough* in 'cough' or that *ou* in 'scout' is pronounced differently in the word 'dough'. With this selection alone it can be seen that sounding out, even if you have learned the 'rules', is certainly not an entirely reliable system.

Another method, and one which tends to make many 'phonics' supporters hot under the collar, is what is sometimes called the 'whole word approach'. This may also be termed the *look and say* method. This involves gaining a visual picture of the word rather than relying on the sound of it. Once again this will be successful under some circumstances and with some learners but will not be adequate for all situations, particularly those times when a reader meets a word that has never been encountered before. *The key is for learners to be able to freely access a range of strategies which make sense to them and which work for them. It would certainly be a mistake for a parent or teacher or tutor to go full steam ahead with one or another approach and then assume there must be something wrong with the learner if the desired effect isn't achieved.*

Seeking Help
Throughout his school years John's parents sought help for him from a range of people. Some of these were of more help than others. Finding the right person can be a confusing and expensive undertaking because of the individual nature of learning difficulties. As has already been stated—there is no one dyslexic condition, therefore there is no one solution. What may work admirably for one person may have no beneficial effect on another.

In an effort to assist in the process of seeking help, here is an outline of some of the professionals who offer services in the area of learning difficulties. Some work only in this field, but most offer help within a broader practice. These are not listed in order of priority:

1 *Educational Field*
  (i) Regular Teachers—The student's regular teachers would be the first point of contact in seeking assistance. They are likely to have a broad understanding of the student's strengths and weaknesses. The difficulty is that they may only have limited time to give the additional assistance that may be required. It is always worth discussing your concerns with them and seeking advice on ways in which home and school work together can help the learner.

(ii) Specialists within Schools—If you are lucky enough to have access to specialist staff, they may be able to offer the regular, intensive, focused help that will enable the learner to develop the necessary skills. The disadvantages may include resistance on the part of the learner, having to attend a different class, or being in any way singled out for special attention while at school.

(iii) Private Tutors—The level of expertise among tutors can vary from highly-qualified specialists, trained to work with areas of learning disability, to under-graduate students, who are able to help with specific subjects, but are not learning experts. Even among the former, strategies may vary widely, with some maintaining a strong affiliation to one particular teaching/learning method, to the exclusion of others. For example, there still exists considerable disagreement among some professionals regarding the value of taking a phonic approach to teaching spelling. I am inclined to advise you to beware of any expert claiming to have THE solution. What is needed is an eclectic approach, which can draw from a number of strategies, depending upon the needs of the learner.

2 *Medical Field*
(i) General Practitioners and Paediatricians— Often, if a child is not succeeding in school, a medical opinion will be sought. Naturally, the advice and strategies offered from this source will tend to focus on organically based problems within the learner, in the expectation that the

learning difficulty will be alleviated through the detection and treatment of such a problem. Attention-Deficit Disorder is a recognised medical condition which may result in learning problems, and which has proven responsive to medication. By providing a thorough physical check, doctors can confirm or eliminate the possibility that illness is a source of the learning problem.

(ii) Psychologists—There is a wide variety of services offered within this field. Some psychologists rely upon the administration of various standardised tests, to determine whether there may be problems in important learning areas, such as auditory memory or visual memory. They can then offer advice in terms of strategies based upon the information provided by the tests. This may be able to be implemented within the regular learning environment, or may require additional tutoring sessions.

Other psychologists may take an approach which seeks an explanation for the learning difficulty within the family relationships or as a result of past or continuing stress or trauma, to which the learner may have been exposed. Counselling may then be offered as a means of dealing with the problems.

3 Other Medical Services

(i) Speech Therapists—Where there is any indication of speech problems, speech therapy may be an essential strategy on which later remediation techniques can be built. There is considerable evidence to suggest that incomplete language acquisition can inhibit the successful learning of reading and spelling, and it is important that this be attended to as early as possible.

(ii) Optometrists—Checking eyesight is, of course, another essential consideration. This needs to be a comprehensive examination, as problems with binocular vision would not be noticed with simple eye checks, and correct binocular vision is essential for ease of reading (as is clear vision for reading books relatively close-up, and charts and boards at a distance).

Various experts have noted eye tracking difficulties or faulty eye movements as factors in reading difficulty; there is some dispute however about which comes first—the eye problems or the reading difficulty.

(iii) Auditory Tests—These will probably have been done when the child was a baby, and, hopefully, any problems will have been detected early. Again, if you suspect that your child is not hearing clearly, or seems unable to distinguish certain sounds, an auditory examination may be warranted.

One form of treatment therapy for dyslexia is the result of an inner ear problem, known as cerebellar-vestibular dysfunction, and is correctable with medication.

4 *Alternative Health Practitioners*
There is a wide range of services available in the field of alternative health and wellness therapies and some have proven helpful in dealing with educational

problems. While this is not a comprehensive list, it would include:

(i) CHIROPRACTORS—By adjusting misalignments of the spinal column, chiropractors have been able to correct various bodily ailments and facilitate more effective working of the entire body systems. It is possible that such treatment could facilitate greater ease of learning if the problems stem initially from structural problems in the body. There is evidence in the chiropractic literature to support this.

(ii) NATUROPATHS AND HOMEOPATHS—may also have strategies which can be of benefit to some individuals. Nutritional imbalances or food allergies are sometimes implicated in learning difficulties, but again the efficacy of these strategies will depend upon the needs of the individual learners.

Some of these less conventional strategies stimulate a great enthusiasm and publicity initially and then seem to die a natural death or are debunked in a hail of negative publicity. The problem seems to lie in the desire that people have for a universal cure for problems like dyslexia. Thus a strategy which has worked successfully for some individuals is picked up by the media and promoted widely. However, when it doesn't work for everyone, it is then dismissed as a fraud. But the truth is that it is neither a 'cure', nor a 'fraud'; it is simply appropriate and successful for some cases but not for all.

What must be taken into account is that overcoming the underlying difficulty (if there is one) will not necessarily result in immediate improvements in the reading and writing problem. Naturally, if students have had difficulty learning, for whatever reason, they will still need help to catch up on what they have missed. The sooner any underlying difficulty is recognised and attended to, the better.

5 Irlen Lenses or Coloured Glasses
In the last decade there have been some interesting new developments which have offered hope for helping people with Dyslexia. There is an understandable reluctance on the part of professionals to recommend new therapies and 'solutions', because they may be expensive and there is no guarantee that they will help. However, I will mention 'coloured glasses' as they have attracted considerable public attention and interest.

Helen Irlen, in 1983, identified a collection of perception disorders which she called 'scotopic sensitivity syndrome' as a factor in certain types of reading disabilities. She discovered that by using different coloured lenses to filter light she could improve reading performance in certain individuals. While it has been estimated that 2.7 per cent of school children may be affected by this syndrome, with up to 70 per cent of those who suffer learning difficulties being affected,[6] it has not been conclusively proven through controlled trials coloured lenses are an effective solution. Nevertheless, there is sufficient interest in the possibilities of this form of therapy to warrant the recommendation, in a report commissioned by the Australian Institute of Health, of the implementation of a long term study to investigate the effectiveness of the lenses.

Studies conducted overseas have neither proved nor disproved the effectiveness of the lenses, although one study found that inexpensive coloured overlays in books were at least as effective as expensive coloured lenses.[7]

In John's case, his parents recalled him phoning with excitement to tell them about a program on television which said that these special glasses would make a difference to dyslexics. All the necessary inquiries were made and John was tested and fitted with the glasses, full of hope that they would be successful. However, when asked about them recently, he shrugged and said he never wore them. For someone with John's energy and impatience for results, this may just have been too slow for him to get the result he was so keen to see. Therefore expectations of 'miracles' are likely to produce disappointments which may lead to the judgement that the glasses are useless.

Coloured glasses like all other so called 'cures' are not magical. If the learner has been unable to process the incoming information effectively during his/her schooling then simply correcting the visual problem will not produce an instantly dramatic change in reading and spelling. It may mean that the learner is now in a much better position to begin learning the skills, but there may still be a lot of work to be done to overcome the deficiencies caused by years of restricted learning.

Do you grow out of it?
This is a difficult question to answer. There does not seem to be any indication that, left to their own devices, dyslexic learners will at some point magically throw off the problem. The fact that in many cases the condition is not recognised or acknowledged until the person is an adult, suggests that it is a life

long condition. However we must not fall into the trap of thinking that because a child is having trouble at school they are necessarily dyslexic. Nor should we act as if there is nothing we can do to make a difference. What is clear is that children vary in the ages at which they are ready to begin reading effectively. Some will do so well in advance of commencing school. For others it may not occur until age eight or nine. What is extremely important for this latter group is that they, and those around them, maintain a positive attitude to learning. Enormous harm can be done to a child's self esteem and future ability to learn effectively if too much emphasis is placed on their deficiencies too early.

Having said this, I acknowledge that it is difficult for parents and teachers to know when is the right time to offer the help. All I can say is, there is no formula; each child will be different. Let the child be the guide. Watch, notice, listen and be ready to help when the time is right. Ensure that whoever is helping knows what they are doing and can offer the learner a positive experience that will produce and reinforce success. In the meantime, continue to support them in the things they learn well and build the picture that they are competent and capable learners.

Conclusion

While there are many books, programs, strategies and techniques designed to help overcome learning difficulties, there is also some evidence to suggest that some learners will continue to experience problems, especially in spelling, throughout their lives. Why this should be, we do not know. But what it does indicate is that we need to be aware that an over attentiveness to the mistakes may blind us to the real ideas being expressed.

Thus a program which recognises and values all of a learner's intelligences and, using these as a guide, develops strategies which genuinely match the learner's preferred modes of learning, should not only facilitate more effective learning but contribute to the positive enhancement of the learner's self esteem. By building on the learner's strengths, rather than concentrating on the weaknesses, there is far more scope for the learning process to be enjoyable, relevant, and most importantly, successful.

References

Part 1
1 McCormack, Mil *Exceeding the Limits—Goal Based Assessment in Practice* in Assessment and Learning in English (Victorian Association for the Teaching of English 1984 C. L. Reynolds Ed.)

Part 2
1 Hornsby, Beve *Overcoming Dyslexia* Macdonald and Co. Ltd London, 1984, p. 32

2 Melman, Barbara *Speld News* June 1991, p. 3

3 Cambourne, Brian Beyond the Deficit Theory: A 1990s Perspective on Literacy Failure, *Australian Journal of Reading*, Vol. 30, Nov. 1990

4 Vail, Patricia, Gifts, Talents and the Dyslexias: Wellsprings, Springboards and Finding Foley's Rocks, *Annals of Dyslexia*, Vol. 40, 1990, p. 16

5 Clay, Marie *The Early Detection of Reading Difficulties: A Diagnostic Survey With Recovery Procedures*, Heinemann Educational 1985

Part 3
1 Hampshire, Susan *Susan's Story—An Autobiographical Account of MY Struggle With Dyslexia*, Sidgwick and Jackson Ltd, New York, 1982

2 Gardner, Howard *Frames of Mind. The Theory of Multiple Intelligences*, Basic Books, USA, 1985

3 Vail, Patricia, op. cit. p. 13

4 Grinder, Michael *Righting the Educational Conveyor Belt* Metamorphus Press, Portland, Oregon, 1989

5 Vail, Patricia, op. cit. pp. 8–10

6 Lea, Anthony and Hailey, David *Tinted Lenses in Treatment of the Reading Disabled*, Australian Institute of Health, Health Care technology Series No. 2, Australian Government Publishing Service, Canberra, 1990

7 Cardinal, D. N., Griffin, J. R. and Christenson, G. N. Do Tinted Lenses Really Help Students with Reading Disabilities?, *Intervention in School and Clinic*, Vol. 28, No. 5 May 1993

Additional Reading

Armstrong, Thomas *In Their Own Way—Discovering and Encouraging Your Child's Learning Style*, Jeremy P. Tarcher Inc., Los Angeles, 1987

Dennison, Paul E. and Gail E. *Brain Gym*, Edu-Kinesthetics Inc., California, 1989

Jensen, Eric *Superteaching* (Master Strategies for Building Student Success), Turning Point, Del Mar, California, 1988

Lazear, David *Seven Ways of Teaching* (The Artistry of Teaching with Multiple Intelligences), Skylight Publishing, Illinois, 1991

Lazear, David *Seven Ways of Knowing* (Understanding Multiple Intelligences), Skylight Publishing, Illinois, 1991

Markova, Dawna *How Your Child is Smart*, Conari Press, Berkeley, California, 1992

Parker, A & Cutler-Stuart, M *Switch On Your Brain*, Hale & Iremonger, Sydney, 1986

Pheloung, Barbara and King, Jill *Overcoming Learning Difficulties*, Doubleday Australia, 1992

Sasse, Margaret *If Only We'd Known*, Toddler Kindy Gymbaroo, Victoria, Australia, 1979

Storz, Moni Lai *Mind Body Power—The Self Help Book On Accelerated Learning*, Time Books International, Singapore, 1989

Vitale, Barbara Meister *Unicorns Are Real* (A Right Brained Approach to Learning), Jalmar Press, California, 1982

Index

Ability, 19, 23
Accelerative learning, 91
aggression, aggressive, 15, 22
Anxiety, 18
Attention Deficit Disorder (ADD), 98
Authority, 21

Bandler, Richard, 77
brain, *vii*, 42, 68, 69, 91

Cambourne, Brian, 45–46
cerebellar vestibular dysfunction, 99
coloured glasses, 11, 101–102
colour, 85

Dennison, Dr Paul E, 68
Dyslexia, dyslexic, *vii*, 1–4, 6–7, 11, 34, 38, 69, 71, 73, 75, 101, 103

Educational Kinesiology, 68
English, 9, 12, 26–27, 48, 57, 61
examinations, 26, 63

failure, 16, 50–51, 58, 61, 84–85
frustration, 3, 14, 15, 33, 35, 36, 43, 50, 84, 86

Gardner, Dr Howard, 73–76
Grinder, John, 77
Grinder, Michael, 77

Hampshire, Susan, 70
Hinshelwood, James, 67

Intelligences, 73–76, 78, 104
Irlen, Dr Helen, 101–102

Kinesthetic learning, 73, 75, 77–78, 81

learning
  auditory, 76–81, 90
  by doing, 31, 32, 33, 49, 71, 80, 81
  kinesthetic, 73, 75, 77–78, 81
  strengths and weaknesses, 47
  -styles, 74 80, 86, 94
  visual, 76–81, 88
literacy, 44, 45

movement and learning, 33, 42, 80
music, 73–75, 85, 91

Neurolinguistic Programming, 77, 89

Orton, Samuel, 68

phonics, 93–95
physical education, 16, 32–33, 56, 58, 63
physical fitness, 56
psychology, psychologists, 98

remedial classes, 12
respect, 15, 54

scotopic sensitivity syndrome, 101
self esteem, 7, 11, 36, 47, 50, 75, 104
speech, 43–44
speech therapy 51, 98
spelling, 59, 62, 63, 70, 88–90, 92–93, 104
sport, *vii*, 55, 56, 62
stress, 84
suggestion 92
Suggestopedia, 91

testing, psychological, 11, 24, 55, 98
tutors, tutoring, 29, 45, 46, 48, 51, 75

Vail, Patricia, 47, 73, 82
visualization, visualizing, 32

word blindness, 67–68, 70